# What *No One* Tells You About Pregnancy

## *What you don't Expect When You're Expecting a Baby*

A Sincere Guide on Emotions and Your Body's Changes During Pregnancy

## Anne Mary Holmes

# Table of Contents

# Introduction

Hello there, mama to be!

First, congratulations on your pregnancy. Having a baby for the first time is one of the most exciting things that can happen to you as a woman. However, there are mixed feelings that you will have to deal with since you may not know what to expect. Maybe you have been planning this pregnancy for years now or it happened to you unexpectedly. Whatever the case, you should prepare yourself for a wonderful experience. Since this little one will be your first baby, expect to be filled with lots of uncertainty. Thankfully, this is normal. There are plenty of questions that you will ask yourself within the next nine months. Your body will go through numerous changes and you will want to know what's going on.

Everyone will be there by your side trying to advise you on what you should be doing. "Eat this, eat that, do this, don't do that." With advice coming from everyone, you can't be sure what's right. There is also plenty of information on the internet concerning pregnancy. You have the freedom of watching videos, reading books and magazines, etc. to equip yourself with the knowledge you require to move from the first trimester to the last safely. Without a doubt, with all this information all around you, it is daunting to know what to do as people offer varying advice concerning pregnancy. Therefore, it is imperative to have accurate information.

With reliable information at your disposal, you will be in a better position to make sound decisions about taking care of yourself and your baby.

This manual compiles all you need to know about pregnancy. It strives to make sure that you go through a successful and happy pregnancy. The information detailed in this guide will guarantee that you know what to expect during the entire period that you will be taking care of your baby before introducing him/her to this world.

A healthy pregnancy also means taking care of your emotional wellbeing. You can't go through a healthy and happy pregnancy if you struggle to keep your emotions in check. Having a baby for the first time is significant. As a result, you should expect a big transformation in your life. Surprisingly, this happens right after you learn that you're pregnant. You will have to make numerous changes from that point on that will make sure you and your baby are safe. For example, if you are an outgoing person, you may have to tone down your extravagant and busy lifestyle for the benefit of you and your baby's health. Similarly, for optimal health during and after pregnancy, maintaining a balanced diet is important.

Along with good health, the support that you get from friends and family will make a huge difference throughout your pregnancy journey. For example, the emotional support you get will strengthen you to overcome anxiety associated with labor. In the long run, your family and friends will be there to help you and support you raise your child. This book will also benefit your partner, friends, and family. Share this with them to help them understand all there is to know about pregnancy. This will be helpful as they will know what to do when you need help from them, and you will all be on the same page when it comes to making decisions.

One of the most distinct aspects of this book is that it offers you an in-depth analysis of everything that will happen at every stage of your pregnancy, on a week-by-week basis. This will help clear up any uncertainties that you might have concerning the emotional and physical changes that you will be going through. What's more, you will also garner up-to-date information about exercise, nutrition, antenatal care, and preparing yourself for labor.

Sometimes there are complications associated with pregnancy. These complications are also discussed in this book to ensure that you know how to deal with them. In addition, there are also a few portions that will discuss your relationship with your partner and how you can take care of your baby together. There are emotional changes that you will experience from time to time. As a result, it is essential that you know how to adjust without affecting your relationship with your partner.

Let's also not forget those who might not be pregnant yet but are planning a pregnancy. If this is the case for you, then this book will still be a valuable companion. Learning more about pregnancy psychologically prepares you to understand that it's not as scary as most people believe. What's more, by getting the facts right about pregnancy, you will be better equipped to make the right decisions on whether it's the right step for you and your partner to take.

If you have plans to get pregnant soon, it is imperative that you talk to a doctor, nurse, or midwife for preconception advice. Moreover, your doctor should also conduct a health check-up to confirm whether there are health problems that could affect your pregnancy. For instance, high blood pressure, depression, epilepsy, and diabetes can pose a threat to you and your unborn baby. Your general practitioner should also talk to you about the importance of having a dental check-up. These factors and many more are some of the things that you should consider when preparing to conceive a baby. More about this will be discussed in detail in this guide.

Now, read on for a comprehensive look into your pregnancy as a first-time mom.

# Part 1: The First Trimester

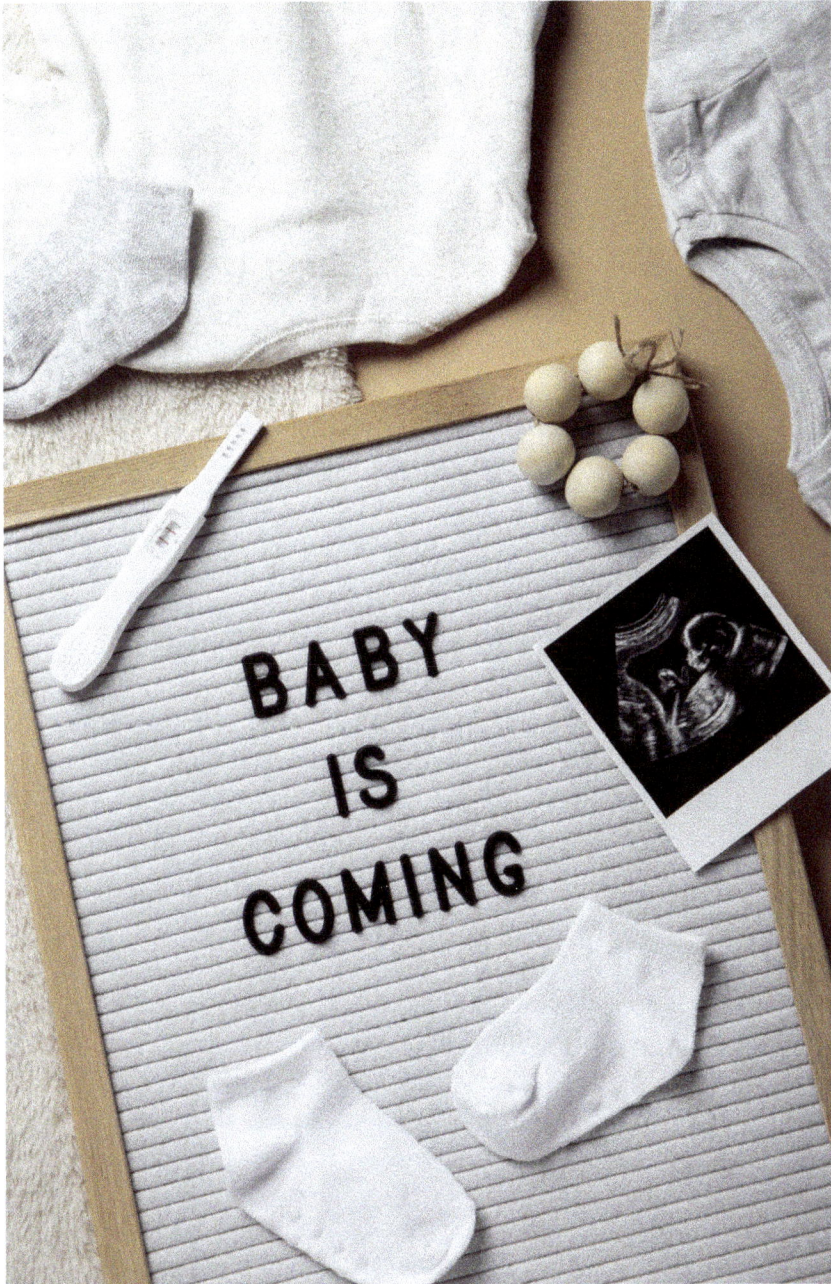

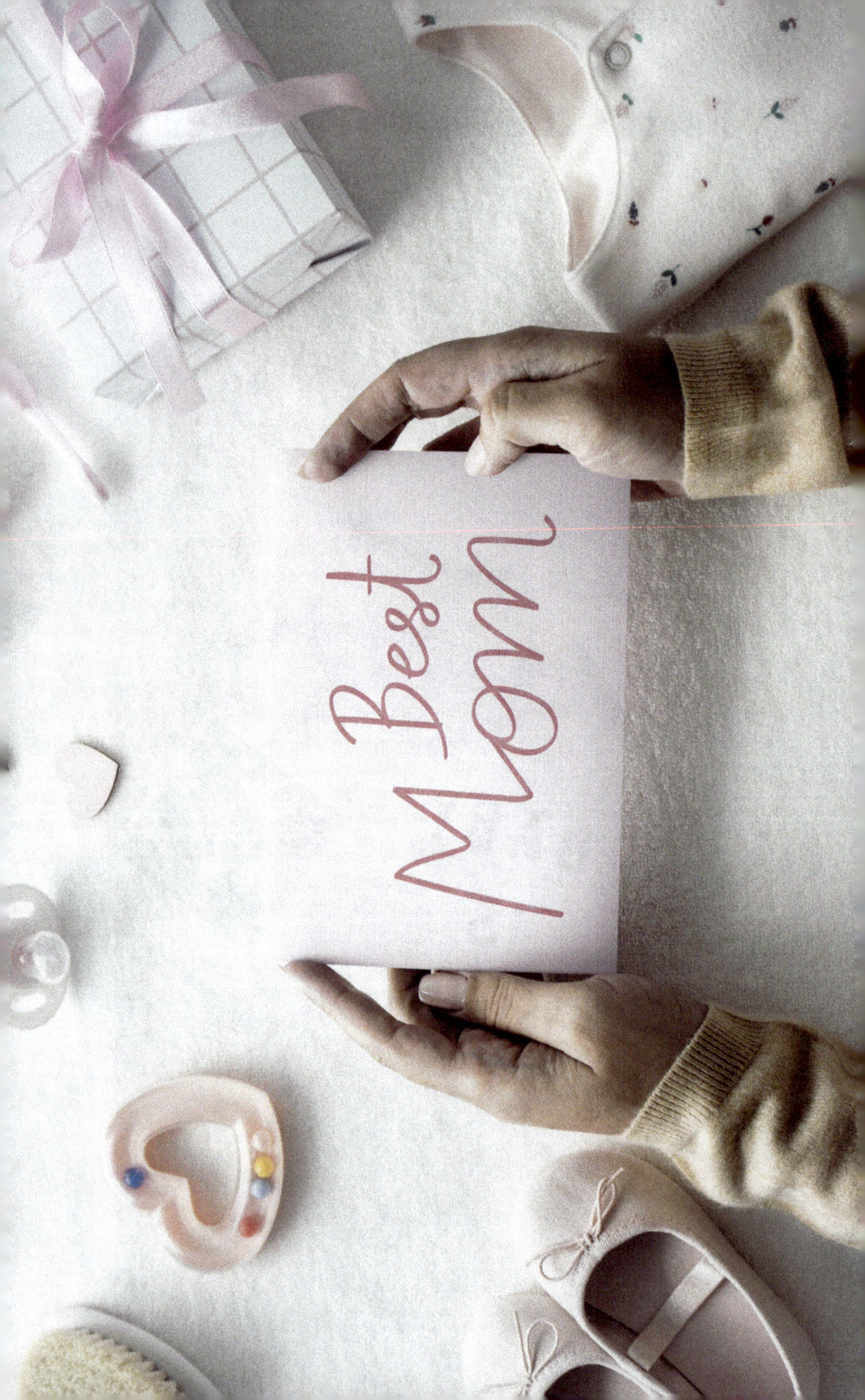

# Chapter 1: Pleasure and Panic When You See the Plus Sign on the Test

You've done everything you can to get and stay healthy—to prepare your body to carry your baby. You've been charting and checking your basal temperature regularly. You've been stuffing those sheets for a few months or more. You've been waiting patiently. You've been keeping up with a healthy lifestyle—exercising and eating right, taking your vitamins, and finding ways to relax. What else can you do?... Wait.

It comes about time for your period to hit. You wait. It's a day late, maybe two. You start to get excited, but no... You have all the symptoms of your period starting soon. You have had for a few days now. Your breasts are tender. You're tired. You're crampy. You're bloated. You're having mood swings. Your back hurts. You're even craving chocolate! Surely, you'll be starting soon. You wait a few more days. Still nothing.

You start to get nauseous. The thoughts of certain foods start to make you sick. There are specific smells that make you want to puke. You start to wonder, but you've wondered every month. You've taken so many tests that you're nickeling and diming yourself to death. Do you really want to put your emotions on the line again? To put yourself through that again. You're about to give up. It seems like it's taking forever. Will this miracle ever happen?

Finally, four days after your period's due, your husband

prompts you to test. It doesn't take much prompting. You're getting excited yourself. I mean four days late. Nausea? Aversion to food? Surely this is it! ...or is it... I mean the flu is going around at the office.

All you think about at work all day long is buying that test. You almost miss the meeting with your manager late that morning. You whisper the news to your best friend over your lunch break while you're both standing at the water cooler. She squeals and practically jumps up and down. That's when you realize that the whole department will know about the possibility by the end of the day. What a mistake you've made! ...but you find you don't care!

After work, you virtually skip into the pharmacy. You can't wait until morning to test, but you bide your time. You try to keep yourself busy. You clean the house, dusting the already clean coffee table and mantel, washing the mirrors, leaving streaks in your haste, and folding neglected laundry. Hey! At least it's clean!

You can't sleep. Come morning, 5:30 am, you jump out of bed.

Good enough. You grab your pregnancy test, sit on the toilet, and read the package once more. You want to make sure you do this right. You should be a pro by now. After all, you've done this every month for four months.

Your hands shaking, you pee in the little Dixie cup you've grabbed from the cupboard under the sink, filling it a little less than half full. Your hands shaking, you pull it out and set it on the floor. You carefully pick up the test you have opened and sitting within reach on the fluffy, dark green rug sitting in front of the bathroom sink on top of the wrapper it came out of and with that on top of the box. You carefully pick that up and hold the absorbent tip in your urine for five seconds.

You can't help but stare at the little window. Almost immediately, the display reads, "YES!" You squeal out loud, almost a scream. You hear your husband's coffee cup slam to the table, his chair knock over backward, clattering to the floor, and him running through the house. He runs into the bathroom, slamming open the door, banging it off the wall.

His eyes are wide as saucers. His face is pale. His breathing is hard and coming in gasps. "Are you okay?" he asks. He starts to calm down as he sees you sitting safely on the toilet with a big smile spread across your face instead of sprawled out on the floor, head gashed open from a nasty fall. He takes a deep breath and shakes his head, presumedly to clear his mind. "Are you okay?" he repeats himself, much calmer this time.

You turn the pregnancy test around slowly so he can see the "YES" in the window.

His face changes from one of annoyance to one of unbelief and to one of pure joy. He takes a few steps forward and pulls the test toward himself so he can get a better look, nearly kicking the cupful of pee over (That would've been bad!). A smile spreads across his face. His face turns a ruddy red as he seems to consider what this means.

"Do you think it'll be a boy?" he asks, his smile growing bigger.

You smile at his eagerness. "I don't know, Honey."

He peeks at his watch. He looks a second time, this time for longer. His eyes get big. "I've got to run!" he half shouts. "I'm late!" He starts to turn, turns back for a kiss, looks at the test one more time, and rushes out the door.

You sigh deeply. You're starting out on a brand-new journey. You are positive.

# Chapter 2: Who Do You Tell, When and How?

The timing of the big reveal is very personal. Some people like to announce their pregnancy as soon as the pee dries on the pregnancy test, and some wait until they can't possibly hide it anymore. Between those two ends of the spectrum, many choose to announce their pregnancy toward the end of the first trimester or the beginning of the second trimester once they've had one or two ultrasounds.

No matter what time feels more comfortable to you to let the world in on your huge secret, there are fun and cute ways you can make the announcement. A simple search for "pregnancy announcement" on Pinterest will take you to what seems like endless options and ideas. Keep in mind that no matter how you choose to tell the world, your inner circle will definitely appreciate hearing it from you in person rather than seeing it on social media (more on that later). That said, here are a few of my favorites:

• The flat lay photo. Spell out all the details on a letter board or with chalk on a blackboard, arrange cute baby things around it, and take a photo from directly above. Send the photo by text and e-mail and post it on social media.

• The hidden-message photo. Take a photo of your favorite spot in the house with a pacifier in the foreground, or a picture of your dog bringing you a tiny pair of shoes.

Say nothing else when you share it and see how long it takes people to pick up on its real meaning.

- The family videoconference call. This is especially great when you have family spread out all over the place. Use a group videoconferencing service to get everyone on your computer screen at once. Then none of them can be upset that they found out after someone else. Plus, you'll have the option of recording their reactions.

- The personal gift. Tell baby's grandparents by gifting them a box of small baby items—think pacifiers, blankets, small toys—to keep at their house for future visits.

- The telling tee. Casually walk into a family dinner rocking a "Does this shirt make me look pregnant?" tee, or something equally telling. No need to figure out what to say. Let the shirt do the work for you and be sure your partner is ready with the camera to get video and photos of people's reactions.

If grand gestures really aren't your thing, that's fine, too. A pregnancy announcement doesn't count any less if you simply call people up and tell them the good news. I encourage you to share the news in person or over the phone first with close family and friends before sharing social media announcements with the world. This seems to matter a lot, especially to the older generation, who aren't so down with the idea of getting major announcements from those they love via their newsfeed so please be patient and mindful with them.

# Chapter 3: The Fear and the Facts of Miscarriage

Antenatal fetal death is an intrauterine fetal death during pregnancy with a gestational age of 8 to 42 weeks.

## *Causes*

Intrauterine fetal death can occur under the influence of various external and internal factors. Pathology can occur on the basis of such endogenous factors as infectious diseases (tuberculosis, viral hepatitis, rubella virus), somatic diseases (heart failure, heart defects, kidney abnormalities, respiratory failure, anemia, kidney disease, endocrine system dysfunction and diabetes mellitus.

In addition, endogenous causes of antenatal fetal death include gestosis, severe fetal developmental pathologies incompatible with life, incompatibility of blood groups or Rhesus conflict between the mother and the fetus, low and high water levels, circulatory disturbance in the placenta, true umbilical cord nodule, inflammatory damage to the female genital organs, entwining the umbilical cord of the fetus. Among other, possible causes of antenatal fatal death.

Exogenous agents capable of provoking fetal death during gestation include intoxications due to poisoning by alcohol, drugs, household, or industrial toxic substances. Also, such pathological processes can be associated with irradiation with ionizing radiation or traumatic damage to the abdomen. In some cases, fetal death occurs for unknown and uncontrollable reasons.

### Symptoms

In the event of fetal death, the uterus ceases to increase in size. Fetal movements disappear, uterine tone decreases or rises. The elasticity of the mammary glands is reduced. Sometimes a woman's general well-being may worsen, and unreasonable weakness appears, pulling pains in the lower abdomen.

Also, the absence of a heartbeat indicates the death of the fetus. From 9 to 10 weeks, the absence of heart contractions is established during ultrasound examination, from 13 to 15 weeks during electrocardiography or phonocardiography of the fetus, and from 18 to 20 weeks during auscultation. In the absence of cardiac contractions in the fetus, an ultrasound examination, cardiography and a blood test for hormones can additionally be prescribed.

### Treatment

If fetal death occurs in the first trimester, a miscarriage may occur. If a miscarriage does not occur, the patient undergoes a medical abortion. In the case of fetal death in the second trimester of gestation, self-expulsion of the fetus is very rare, because of which an urgent delivery is carried out. A woman undergoes labor excitement. For this, a woman is shown the introduction of estrogen, glucose, vitamins, and calcium preparations, after which the administration of oxytocin and prostaglandins is carried out.

In the case of fetal death in the third trimester, independent births sometimes occur. If labor is absent, then they are stimulated or might undergo an operation.

### Prevention

Prevention of antenatal death is based on the timely detection of genetic abnormalities, the treatment of somatic diseases, the rehabilitation of the foci of infection, the rejection of bad habits and the cessation of contact with household toxic substances.

Note: Do remember that no matter what happens no one wants it to happen, especially you. Mothers tend to blame themselves, but it is never their fault. In reality it is no one's fault. Things just really happen.

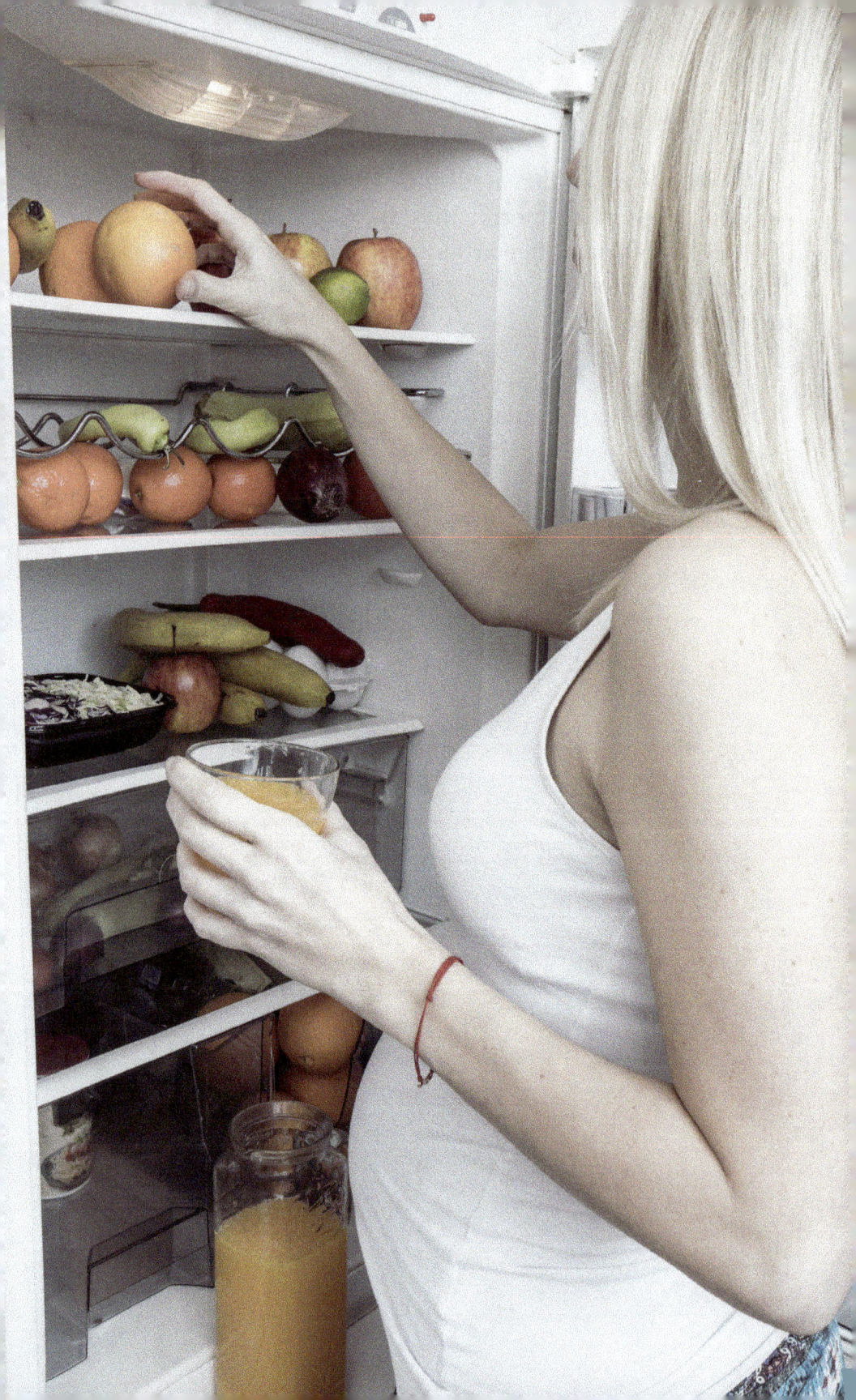

# Chapter 4: Nutritional Issues During the First Trimester

## *Morning Sickness*

Nausea does influence about half experience vomiting and most pregnant women as well while not everyone suffers from morning sickness. The fantastic thing is however if you are the person that may seem like an eternity that morning sickness subsides after the first trimester. Specific eating habits can make a difference, while few medications are readily available to assist. Food might be the last thing you want when eating small amounts frequently, although feeling nauseous is vital to observe -- an empty belly makes nausea worse in people. Not to mention you need to be taking your baby needs.

Stay away from the temptation. They're a snack that is convenient but is not rich in the nutrients. Attempt dried wholegrain crackers and cheese, or nuts and fruit, a bowl of breakfast cereal instead.

There is some evidence that ginger and vitamin B6 may help to decrease nausea -- make certain to discuss this with your GP, midwife, or pharmacist to be sure the amount is safe.

If you aren't managing to keep any food or fluids, see your GP. You may have a condition called hyperemesis gravidarum, which is vomiting severe enough to treat you getting dehydrated. It is uncommon but may require hospital treatment to provide fluids using a drip.

Top 10 Ways to Overcome Morning Sickness

• Begin the day with a snack before you get out of bed. You could keep a box of crackers from the bed, or maybe your spouse will be considerate enough to bring you tea and dry toast.

• Eat a high carbohydrate snack every hour or so.

• Lessen cooking aromas by opening windows and by means of extractor fans when cooking (simpler said than performed if it is winter). From where food is ready eat in a room that is separate. Choose foods that are cool or cold since these have not as an odor.

• Some people today discover that beverages or foods containing ginger aid to relieve nausea. You could attempt ginger beer (non-alcoholic, naturally), ginger ale, or a stir fry garnished with ginger.

• Avoid eating foods that are greasy since they'll sit in your stomach for longer. Some women feel better if they avoid eating foods that are spicy.

• Make foods that are fast to prepare -- or try to find another person to do it.

• Suck on a piece of lemon or a sour sweet.

• Have a sip of a drink every few moments when feeling nauseous.

• Eat smaller meals but comprise snacks to compensate. Eat more in the times of day when you feel better.

• Do not drink a lot with foods (but balance drinking drinks consistently between meals). This can help prevent you from feeling complete at meals and help with nausea.

## *Food Cravings and Aversions*

People laugh about girls craving mad foods. They are very real while most cravings are not so amusing. From chocolate to pickled onions, when they strike, they may be difficult to resist. Provided that you maintain your overall diet there's no fantastic risk of harm; in fact, aversions to caffeine and alcohol in early pregnancy might be helpful. Giving in to frequent cravings for chocolate or crisps may mean filling up on junk food, with less space left for fare.

In case you plan, you can turn your cravings into something healthful. For example, if you're craving crisps, have a much healthier choice on hand such as crunchy cereal bars, celery and carrot sticks, or breadsticks. This way you'll get fiber vitamins and some vitamins with each crunchy bite. When it is a treat you are after, try berries, dried a jam sandwich, mango, or a berry.

Cravings refer to some desire for meals, but women have an overwhelming desire for substances that are not food, such as washing powder or dirt, fit heads. This is a condition called pica, and unlike food cravings it may be harmful if people eat what they crave. You fear you might not be able to resist them, and in case you have cravings for non-foods like these speak to your GP or midwife.

### *Fatigue*

There is nothing quite as sapping as the fatigue that could descend while pregnant. For a lot of us this is an unavoidable part of becoming pregnant, however sometimes it can be due to anemia -- you will be given a blood test to test for this. Getting enough rest can also be crucial. Is to make sure your diet is best. This can help to maintain energy levels as even as possible.

Be sure that you're eating every couple of hours. Regular meals and snacks are crucial to keeping the human body fueled -- try to include some carbohydrate from grain foods or potatoes, and fruit or dairy foods (milk beverages, yoghurt or fromage frais). Now if you can just find a few minutes to put your feet up...

### *Pregnancy Myth Busters: While I'm pregnant, I Want to Eat Absolutely*

There are numerous stresses during pregnancy, and food is a typical one. Life can get in the way, although Everybody wishes to follow every principle perfectly. You may neglect to take healthy snacks need to trust the snack machine and to work. You may be stuck onto a motorway with no options apart from food. Or you may just have and be distressed to get a piece of chocolate cake. Please be reassured that, if you are taking the recommended vitamin supplements, and are generally currently eating a balanced diet, your body will be getting. The is no problem and is one thing you don't need to feel stressed about.

## *Healthy Habits*

Pregnancy is the perfect time for a diet makeover, not only for when the time arrives to set a wholesome example for your young child and while you are pregnant into breastfeeding, but to take on. Part of this entails adopting habits that promote healthy eating and help maintain energy levels throughout the day. You could even begin by writing down what you eat, and if, for a couple of days. Look through the results and see if there are any changes you can make.

Listed below are a couple of areas:

• Food groups -- look through the food collection information. Are you eating what your body requires?

• Ditch the nonsense thought-- check you are eating sugary or fatty foods. Could some of them be replaced with options that were healthier?

• Start the day with breakfast -- is the meal we bypass, and it is even more unwise during pregnancy. Studies show that people who eat breakfast tend to eat more nutritious diets entire, and pregnancy is the time for that. The same applies to bypass meals that are different -- a constant supply of nourishment is critical.

• Healthy snacks -- as being beneficial or healthy than foods we eat at mealtimes, however this is not the case, we often consider snacks. By choosing from the food groups, and avoiding fatty and fatty foods, snacks can be a part of our daily diet.

### *Best 10 Handbag Bites*

- Cereal bar, or fruit and nut or seed pub

- Oat cakes -- plain or flavored

- Flapjack

- Apple, or some fruit

- Dried fruit

- Nuts -- walnuts, peanuts, Brazil nuts or attempt peanuts

- Wholegrain rice cakes (search for lower-salt forms)

- Mixed seeds such as pumpkin seeds and sunflower seeds -- try the flavored varieties

- Wholegrain crackers Full of jam and peanut butter

- Make your own gourmet trail mix of raisins, dried seeds, cranberries, and nuts

# Part 2: The Second Trimester: Grappling with the Logistics of a Changing Body and Family

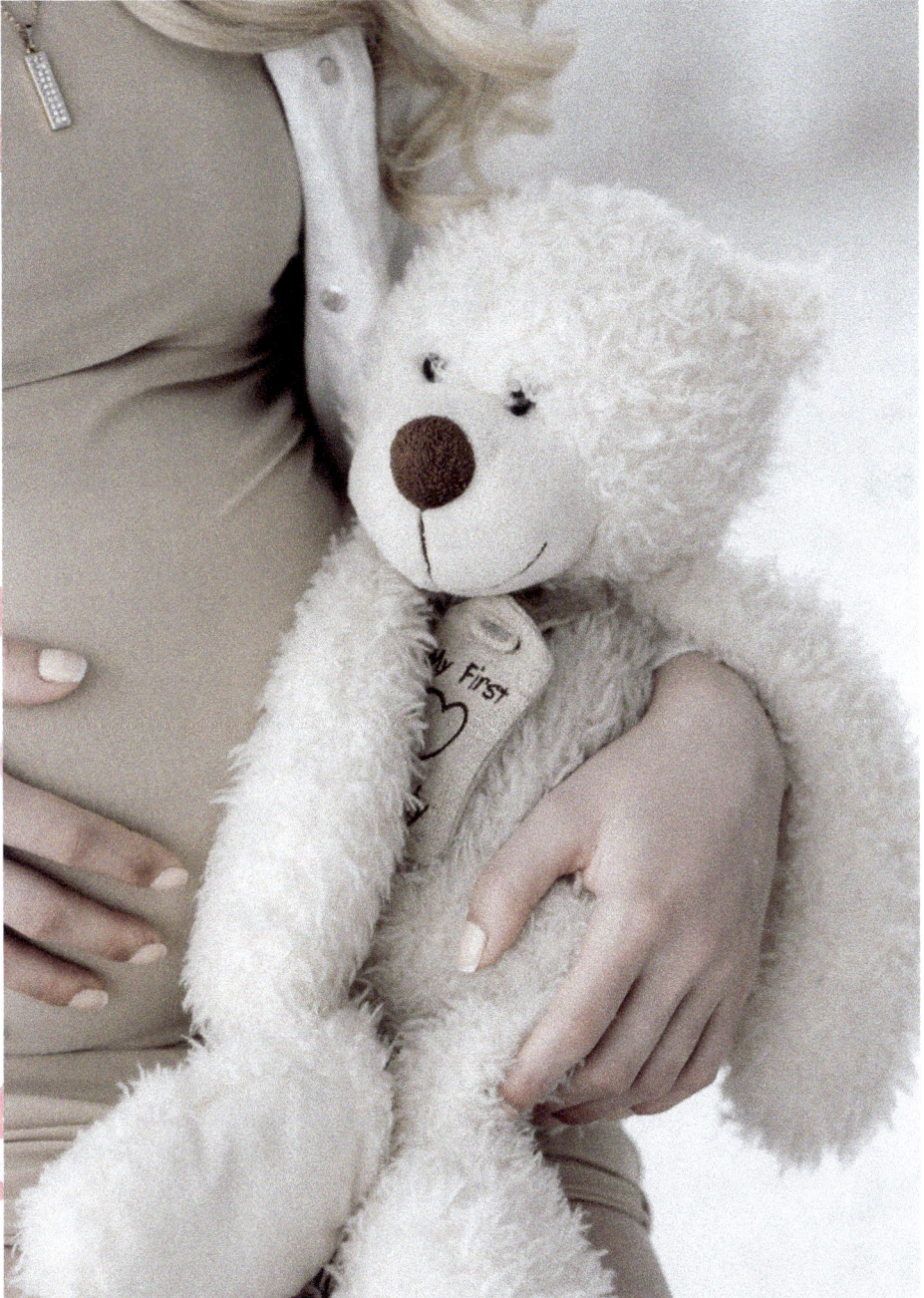

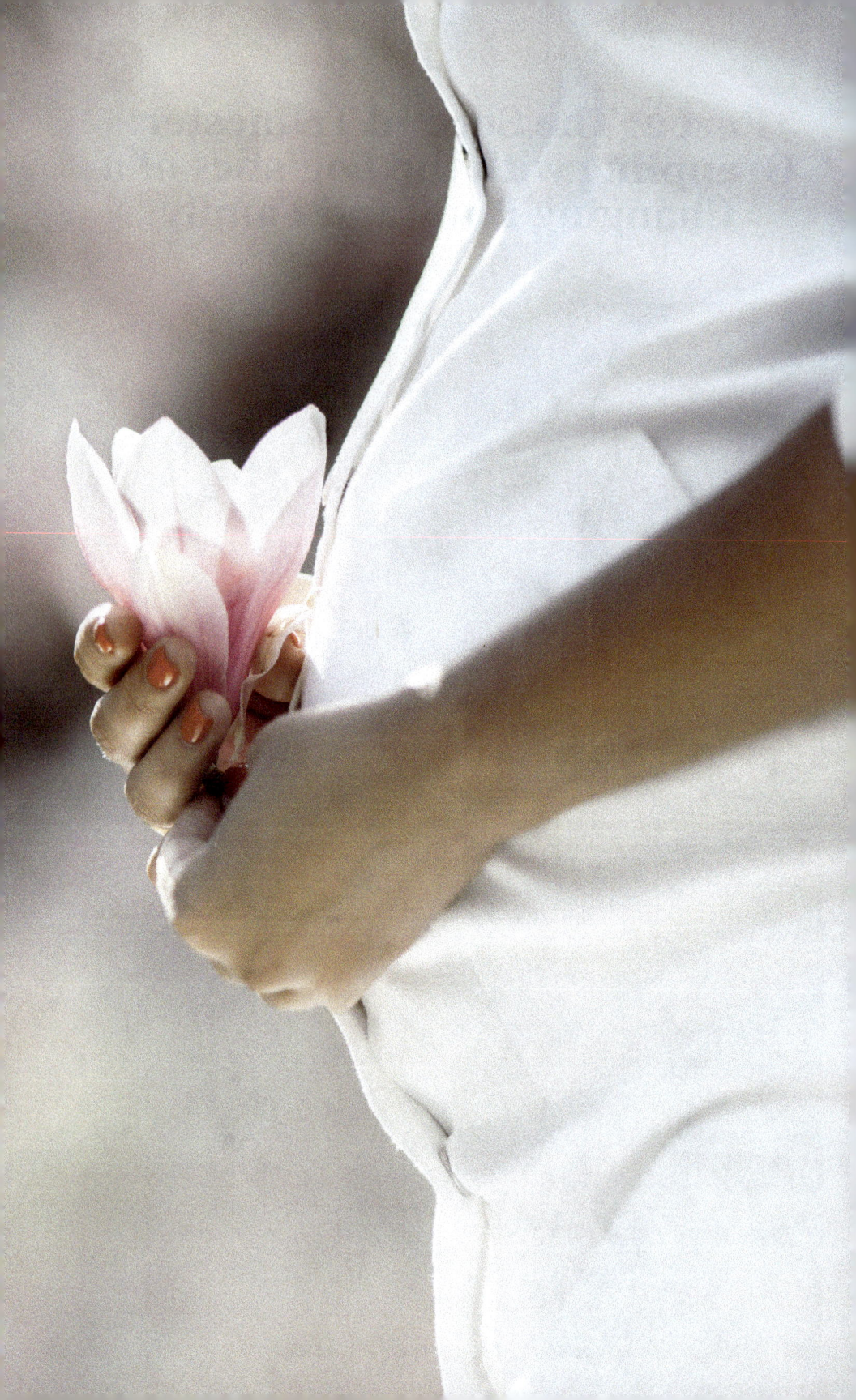

# Chapter 5: Physical and Emotional Changes (Part 1)

Investing in maternity clothes is a sound decision right now. Don't manage your growing abdomen by not buttoning or zipping your pants all the way or employing safety pins to extend your waistband. You will enjoy your pregnancy more with clothing that fits comfortably. Emotionally, you may be feeling scattered and unfocused. You may also be feeling excited, and possibly some misgivings, about "showing."

Now that your early pregnancy symptoms have subsided, you will have more energy and may have more interest in having sex. You may be more likely to have multiple orgasms due to the extra blood flow to the labia, clitoris, and vagina. At the midpoint of your pregnancy, 20 weeks, your uterus measures at the level of your navel so you will need to begin sleeping on your left side. Putting some pillows behind you when you sleep will prevent you from rolling over so you will not lie flat on your back. By the end of the second trimester, your uterus will be about two and a half inches above your belly button, and you will have healthily gained about 19 pounds.

### How's My Pregnancy?

In your second trimester, your practitioner will check on your weight, blood pressure, and the fetal heartbeat. A quad screen, while not conducted on all pregnant women, measures alpha-fetoprotein, hCG, unconjugated estradiol, and inhibin-A levels to determine the presence of Down syndrome. Your practitioner will also conduct a urinalysis and manually evaluate the size of your uterus.

You may have several practical concerns about your pregnancy ranging from how your behavior affects your baby's development to the changing dynamics between you and your partner. Keep a list of the questions, symptoms, and challenges you are experiencing so you can discuss them at each appointment. If you are nervous, or unsure if something is important or serious during your pregnancy, just ask.

Don't be embarrassed! It's better to ask questions, even if only for your own peace of mind. A good provider will take the best possible care of you and your baby. He or she will honor any preferences you have if they are reasonable and workable. That said, get ready to be flexible. There will be much about your pregnancy and birth that you can't predict, but preparing in a healthy way and advocating for what you do want will go a long way toward keeping your pregnancy and delivery smooth and setting your mind at ease.

Even though you are taking a prenatal vitamin, you may still develop iron deficiency anemia during pregnancy as your baby uses some of the iron stored in your body. Iron is the most important supplement to take during pregnancy, so be sure to take a prenatal vitamin that contains iron.

Sign up for childbirth classes if possible, practice your childbirth preparation exercises, and become familiar with the birth process. This is also the perfect time to think about hiring a doula to be your labor support specialist. Your doula can help you plan an advanced tour of the facility where you will deliver your baby and help you choose the appropriate childbirth education classes. Your doula can help you devise your birth plan and help you carry it out. Besides learning childbirth techniques, sign up for an infant CPR and first-aid class. There is no time like the present to keep your newborn safe and sound.

### The Aches and Pains

Growing a baby inside you is a lot of work, and rarely comfortable. You expect that labor and delivery will be painful, but what is happening to you right now? Your body is changing in many ways and in many directions, all at the same time. As your baby grows and develops, your uterus does, too. This means back, abdomen, groin, and thigh aches and pains accompany all the other "joys" of pregnancy. As your baby grows, the pressure of its head, your increased weight, and the loosening of your joints can contribute to backaches and pain near your pelvic bone. If the uterus pinches the sciatic nerve you may experience shooting pain that runs from the lower back down the back of one leg. If this is your first pregnancy, your baby's growth and the resulting discomfort may be surprising. Sometimes the pain will be agonizing; however, safe options for pain relief are available. Here are some treatments for the common aches and pains of the second trimester.

### Heartburn

Heartburn, that burning feeling in your throat and chest, is a symptom of indigestion. It happens as hormones relax the smooth muscle tissue in your gastrointestinal tract. While uncomfortable for you, heartburn benefits your baby. Slower digestion improves the absorption of nutrients into your bloodstream through the placenta and on to your baby. In addition, the hormones responsible for your frequent heartburn, relaxing and progesterone, also cause fetal hair growth, so it's likely that if you're having a lot of heartburn your baby will be born with a full head of hair. Instead of eating three large meals, opt for five or six smaller, balanced, nutritious ones to feel better. In addition, any food that triggers heartburn should be taken off the menu for now. Spicy foods, fried foods, fatty foods, highly seasoned foods, chocolate, mint, coffee, carbonated beverages, and processed meats are likely offenders. Also, keep some sugarless chewing gum in your purse or handbag and try using it about 30 minutes after eating. The act of chewing reduces excess acid by triggering a digestive response.

### Round Ligament Pain

Equivalent to "growing pains," round ligament pain is the result of the stretching of muscles and ligaments that support your growing uterus. It may show up as unilateral sharp, stabbing cramps or dull abdominal aches upon rising from a seated position or when you cough. To relieve and prevent these pains, try to avoid abrupt changes in position. When you move, turn your entire body rather than just turning at your waist. Bending toward the pain will also help relieve the sensation. Even though this symptom is physiologically common, mention it to your provider at your next visit.

### Stretch Marks

During pregnancy, stretch marks may appear on your breasts, abdomen, hips, and buttocks. Gaining weight gradually is the best way to help minimize the marks. You can also promote skin elasticity with a balanced diet rich in vitamin C. After pregnancy, the marks will fade, but they will not disappear; however, there is no harm in applying moisturizers. Avoid steroid creams, as you will absorb them into your bloodstream, and they can pass on to your developing baby. There are no miracle creams that prevent stretch marks. The only treatments for stretch marks, laser therapy and prescriptions containing glycolic acid, can be implemented after pregnancy.

### Leg Cramps

Nighttime calf cramps can disrupt your much-needed sleep. Before going to bed, try stretching your legs first. If cramps still wake you up, massage your calf with long, downward strokes. Straighten your leg and slowly flex your entire foot toward your nose. When possible, avoid standing for long periods and wear compression stockings during the day. You can also use a heating pad on the affected calf, but do not use it for longer than 15 minutes at a time. For severe and persistent cramps, contact your practitioner to rule out the emergent possibility of blood clot formation.

### Dental Issues

Pregnant women are at increased risk for cavities and gum disease. Your gums may swell and bleed due to pregnancy hormones but continue brushing and flossing as usual. Mouthwash and gargles are fine to use. Switching to a softer toothbrush may help your gums feel less irritated. If you have a dentist appointment already scheduled, keep it. A dental checkup in pregnancy ensures that your mouth is healthy. If you need local anesthesia or dental x-rays, let your dentist know that you are pregnant so they can protect your thyroid with a shield. As always, consult your provider before taking any medications.

### *The Best Exercises*

Exercise not only affects your health, but also the health of your developing baby. For low-risk pregnancies, exercise or be active for a total of 30 minutes each day. Working out while pregnant also gives you a head start in getting your body back after delivery. A light exercise and stretching routine in the second trimester can help alleviate a host of conditions and assist in proper fetal positioning, which makes birth easier. If your pregnancy is high risk or if you have had several miscarriages, discuss exercise with your provider before starting an activity. Listen to your body; it will tell you when it is time to slow down. Due to your growing uterus, your body is heavier, and this will ultimately affect your sense of balance. Keep these changes in mind as you adjust your workouts. Here are some suggestions for healthy ways to keep active in your second trimester.

### Walking

There is no easier exercise to fit into your schedule than walking. There is also no special equipment necessary (except supportive, comfortable shoes), and you do not need to pay for gym memberships. The best part? All the walking you do throughout the course of your day counts! Whether it is walking to the farmers' market, parking farther away at the store, or the 10 minutes you spend walking the dog, use these situations to your advantage.

The good news is that you can continue walking right up to delivery, and walking will help aid the natural progression of your contractions. If you weren't active before getting pregnant, walking is as involved as you should get with exercise (swimming is also low impact enough to take on). Walking briskly for 30 minutes every day is the quintessential way to incorporate exercise into your lifestyle. Begin slowly with casual strolling before progressing to a brisk pace. Walking alone gives you the opportunity to quiet your mind, and you can also enjoy the additional benefits of forest bathing. If you would rather have company, invite your partner, friends, or colleagues. You can even join a Meetup group for pregnant women. If the weather doesn't cooperate, you can always join the mall walkers.

## Stretches

Stretching is a great way to stay healthy and ward off some nasty aches and pains. Try the following routines to see which work best for you.

### Hip Flexors

1. Face the stairs, using the wall or railing for support.

2. Put one foot on a step and bend your knee while keeping the other leg straight.

3. Lean into your bent leg, keeping your back straight.

4. Feel the stretch in your straight leg.

5. Switch legs and repeat on the other side.

### Psoas Stretch

1. Lie on your back, using pillows to create a diagonal from your lower back to your head.

2. Bend your knees with your heels a foot away from your buttocks, about hip-width apart.

3. With your hands at your sides, rest in this position for 15 minutes.

## Forward-Leaning Inversion

1.Kneel on the edge of the bed.

2.Lower yourself to the floor, resting on your forearms.

3.Let your head hang freely, chin tucked.

4.Slowly sway your hips.

5.Flatten your lower back.

6.Take three deep breaths.

7.Return to the kneeling position.

# Chapter 6: Physical and Emotional Changes (Part 2)

## Common Symptoms

With the second trimester comes a set of new symptoms. Most of the symptoms from your first trimester should start to ease by the time your second trimester starts. Some exceptions to this are cravings, which can continue into the second trimester, and the changes in your body. These changes won't reverse; they'll just keep changing. Here are some of the other symptoms you can expect in the second trimester.

## Skin Pigmentation Changes

Stretch marks are one of the most noticeable skin changes during the second trimester. As your belly starts to grow, your skin will stretch around the belly, back, thighs, and sometimes, breasts. Most women experience stretch marks and they're often considered a mark of being a warrior mother. They're nothing to be ashamed of and they'll give you fond memories of carrying your child. If there is pain associated with the marks, you can use moisturizers to help your skin maintain elasticity.

Another skin change is something called chloasma, or the mask of pregnancy. It's a change in pigment on your face, around your forehead, nose, and cheeks. This is experienced by some pregnant women, and it will fade after the birth of your child. If you feel self-conscious about this mark, you can usually hide it easily with makeup.

One of the most noticeable changes that happen for many women is a dark line that extends vertically across the belly. It goes from your pubic bone to the top of your belly bump. As your belly grows, so too does the line. It's not harmful, and it's not permanent. You'll usually see it from the beginning of the second trimester.

### Braxton Hicks

During the end of your second trimester, you'll start to experience Braxton Hicks. These are false contractions and occur intermittently throughout the second and third trimester. Not everyone will experience them, and even if you do, you may only experience them as a minor fluttering or tightness in your belly.

Braxton Hicks can sometimes be mistaken for labor, especially in the third trimester. However, they're different from true contractions, as they don't grow stronger and in increased frequency as true contractions do. However, if you think your contractions are labor, it's better to be safe than sorry, so call your medical professional.

If your Braxton Hicks are causing you pain, simply changing your position can often help ease the contractions.

### Back Pain

As your belly grows, your lower spine will start to bend a bit forwards, causing some back pain. Unfortunately, the back pain will remain with you throughout the pregnancy as you start to support a growing baby. To help treat your back pain, you can take up light, low-impact exercise. Regular exercise can be very helpful, while bed rest can make your back pain worse. Supportive pillows can also help ease the discomfort as you try to sleep. There are many pregnancy pillows available online, many of which support both your back as well as your belly. Finally, using heat or ice can also help ease the pain.

If your back pain is severe, talk to your doctor. They may refer you to a physical therapist or prescribe you safe pain medications.

## Other Symptoms

- Improvement in energy levels
- Gain one pound per week
- Frequent urination
- Dizziness or lightheadedness due to low blood pressure
- Pregnancy-related congestion
- Leg cramps
- Swollen feet and ankles

### *Maternal Positioning*

Improper seated positions put undue stress on your spine. At home, practice sitting erect, accentuating the curve of your back, with your shoulders rounded backward and your buttocks touching the back of your chair. Hold this position for a few seconds and then slightly relax. To keep your hips at a 90-degree angle, use a footrest to elevate your feet. Use chairs that provide good support with a straight back, arms, and a cushion. For extra support, place a rolled-up towel or a lumbar roll in the hollow of your back. Prolonged sitting may also prove to be troublesome for your back, so avoid sitting in the same position for more than 30 minutes. At work, trade your office chair for a maternity or exercise ball. The maternity ball will comfort and strengthen your lower back while keeping your pelvis open and supported. To be fair, you may not be able to sit comfortably upright without a few practice attempts. To sit properly using the maternity ball, sit so that your feet and the center of the ball make a tripod. A properly inflated ball will be big enough so that your hips are equal to or higher than your knees.

### Gestational Diabetes

If you have not had diabetes before but you develop it during pregnancy, it is called gestational diabetes (GD). During pregnancy, if you produce less insulin or if your body cannot use insulin appropriately, your blood sugar levels will be high. GD develops between weeks 24 and 28, which is why your provider schedules a routine glucose screening test at 28 weeks. You probably won't show any symptoms even if you do develop GD, but you may experience unusual thirst, overabundant urination, and fatigue. Sugar will be detectable in the urine. A glucose tolerance test follows a glucose screening test if the screening test shows high glucose levels. The tolerance test, done while fasting and on an empty stomach, lasts longer, about three hours, and requires four blood samples.

Untreated, GD has serious repercussions for you and your baby, as you both will be exposed to an unhealthy concentration of sugar. You might have excessive amounts of amniotic fluid, which will swell your uterus and can cause premature labor. You may also have a long labor because your baby is large and cannot fit through the birth canal. In this instance, a cesarean delivery will be required. With high blood sugar, you may experience frequent infections of the kidneys, bladder, cervix, and uterus. You can prevent and treat GD by maintaining a healthy weight, both before and during pregnancy, eating a healthy diet, avoiding refined sugar, exercising regularly, and getting enough folic acid from a balanced diet, 0.8 to 1 milligram a day.

## *Dealing with Emotional Changes*

### Negative Body Image

This is one of the most difficult aspects of pregnancy for many women. With the physical changes happening to your body and your mood, it's easy to start having a negative image of your body. Many women struggle with this and feel very uncomfortable in their shifting body. This is especially true as you start experiencing cravings, fatigue, and mood swings. Your aches and pains will all add to this frustration.

Adjusting to your new body is critically important for your own mental wellbeing. There has been considerable research on this. In one study conducted by the University of York focused on the importance of positive body image during pregnancy, researchers studied 600 pregnant women, and their findings supported additional evidence that showed how body image impacts maternal and infant wellbeing before and after birth (University of York, 2019). Because positive body image creates positive wellbeing for both you and your baby, it's important to work through any feelings of negativity about your body. Here's some advice for you and your partner on how to work through these negative feelings:

### Find three things you really like about your body: Writing down the things

you appreciate about your body can help remind you of how strong and resilient it is, and you are. Noticing how beautiful and supportive your body is, and how it's caring for you and your baby, can help improve your body image. Writing it down, along with some positive phrases to remind you, can honestly help you feel better. Anytime you feel low again about your body, just flip back to those written quotes and re-read them.

Consider taking time to get to know your body: Your body is changing, and with it may come feelings of discomfort. Take some time to re-explore your new body and appreciate it. You can do this sexually with a partner, but you can also do this non-sexually. Taking a warm bath, while staying mindful of the feeling of water around you can be helpful in feeling better. Massaging moisturizing lotion into your belly, breasts, arms, hands, and feet can help you feel more connected to your body.

Do some light exercise: Exercise can help you feel better in general, especially when you're down or feeling overwhelmed by negative self-talk. Going for a simple walk in nature can improve your mood, while working your muscles can make you feel generally better about yourself. The exercise you choose doesn't have to be anything intense. It can be a little walk or a bike ride. You could do some yoga, especially prenatal yoga which is crafted for pregnant women.

Take a picture of your baby bump: Some women find this both celebratory and cathartic. It gives them the opportunity to see their body change while also understanding and accepting why it's changing. You've probably seen these pictures online, in which women stand against the same wall in the same position and take a picture every month to show the changes in their body. If this is something you would feel comfortable with, I encourage you to do it. Taking pictures of your body and watching the changes can help you experience the joy of carrying your child, even when things are difficult.

Stop comparing: This is the same advice you would receive if you have body image issues outside of pregnancy. Simply put, stop comparing your body to your "idealized" body image. Instead of looking at models on Instagram and wishing you had their body, focus on the good things your body provides you with. Also, don't compare your body at week 12 with your body before you were pregnant since there are going to be obvious differences. Instead, focus on how the changes you're going through are positive for your baby. Remember, you'll have all the time you need after your baby is born to return to your pre-baby body or accept your new body as it is.

### Depression and Anxiety

We discussed this a little during the first trimester, but this time, I want to talk about the importance of partner support to ease feelings of depression and anxiety in expectant mothers. Women who receive little support from their partners are more likely to experience higher rates of depression and anxiety about the pregnancy (Er et al., 2016). So, it's incredibly important for your partner to support you. If you don't have a partner, then get support from your family and loved ones. They can provide you with help and friendship when you start to worry about your pregnancy.

Support is more than just being there. It's being able to count on your partner to help however they can. It's also about experiencing affection and love and feeling as though you and your baby matter. If your partner can reassure you that they'll be helpful once the baby is born, that can also relieve some of your anxieties. So, if you start to feel low or anxious about your pregnancy, talk to your partner about how they can better support you.

# Chapter 7: What About Pregnancy Sex?

There are many opinions about sex during pregnancy. Some are totally against it while others feel it's okay. What do you think? Pregnancy has surely raised so many questions. It is true that your body undergoes many changes, and yes, emotional fluctuations may have sex seem unpleasant at times, but simply put, it is not wrong to have sex with your partner when you are pregnant. All you need to do is communicate well with him so you both know what your body wants at each time. The truth is many couples report that having sex during pregnancy is still as mind-blowing as honeymoon sex.

## *Changes in Your Body that Affects Sex*

Let us briefly review the different changes your body will go through during each trimester, both physically and emotionally. Then we will see how these changes should affect your sex life.

### First Trimester

It is a known fact that our breasts will be more sensitive, which may be associated with an increase in size causing either increased pleasure or pain. The areolas (dark area around the nipples) will widen and get darker along with your nipples. It's also possible that nausea and body weakness may diminish your sexual appetite.

Lingering orgasms during sex can result in increased tension in your vagina and your clitoris. So, sex may hurt at times and be pleasurable as well at other times.

### Second Trimester

During the second trimester, the vagina and clitoris will naturally experience more lubrication because of enlargement that will be noticed. So, it is natural that more women will feel sexier during this period, no wonder they call it the "honeymoon period" of pregnancy. You will also feel less sick compared to the first trimester. But in case of concerns, please speak to your doctor.

You can also engage in various other kinds of sex acts if you are an adventurous couple. Just make sure that your partner avoids blowing air into your vagina.

### Third Trimester

Some people avoid sex totally during this phase of pregnancy because it is close to their due date. Just remember that sexual orgasm cannot trigger labor if your cervix is not dilated and ready for childbirth. It is true that you may experience contractions during this stage, but it will be occasionally.

Unless your doctor instructs you not to, having sex during this time is not just great but can prepare your vagina for childbirth. Because of increased fatigue, sex may not be as frequent during this time. The mother is also gaining weight, so it is important for you to try out sex positions that will have sex a little less uncomfortable. Remember the mom-to-be should not lie on her back; she requires to be at least leaning to one side.

### *Benefits of Sex During Pregnancy*

1. It makes you feel connected to your partner.

2. Pregnancy sex feels great, it reminds you of honeymoon days, especially during the second trimester.

3. You'll reap some big health benefits — and even ease some pregnancy symptoms like:

- Burn some extra calories

- Lower your blood pressure

- Sleep more soundly

- Ease pain and discomfort

- Improve your immunity

4. Sex during pregnancy can lift your spirits

5. Your baby will benefit because it results in better health for the fetus.

6. It might be a chance for you and your partner to be creative when it comes to sex positions.

7. Sex will boost your chances of a more successful labor.

8. Having sex during pregnancy will surely lead to a better postpartum experience.

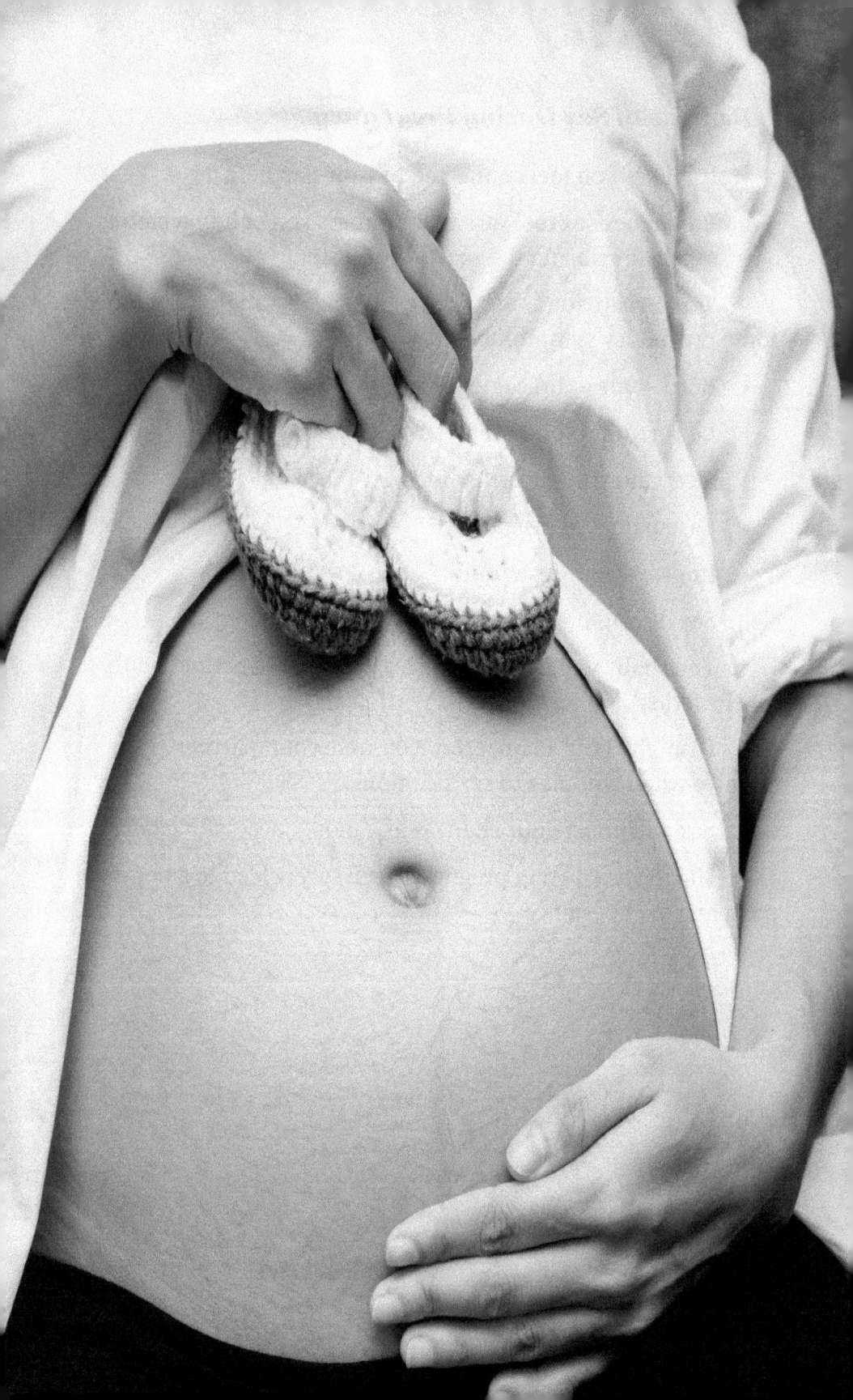

# Chapter 8: The Amazing Effects of Holistic Medicine on Your Pregnancy

The way that you look at childbirth is going to make a huge difference in how you feel during your pregnancy. While the processes of pregnancy and childbirth are physical, there is so much more to the process than that. In fact, they are major transitions in life. You are going from a life without this child to one with this child. Even if you have had children before, your pregnancy will change your life into a 'before' and an 'after.' The changes that are going to occur during pregnancy and the birth of your child will affect every part of your life, including your beliefs, values, and relationships. Therefore, it makes so much sense to use a holistic approach during your pregnancy and consider the spirit, mind, and body.

When you are considering getting pregnant, or if you are already pregnant, you are probably trying to figure out the best things to do to have a healthy pregnancy. You want to know how to have the best emotional and physical health as you possibly can during this time. Many mothers even wonder how they can naturally get through labor without too much pain for themselves or stress to the baby. A holistic approach could be the answer that you need to all these questions and can give you the best pregnancy possible.

### Physical Benefits

First, let's look at some of the physical benefits that you can receive when you use a holistic approach for your pregnancy. Pregnancy is a very physical time. You are growing another human being inside of you. This is going to make some huge changes to your body, both those that can be seen, such as your growing belly and swollen ankles, and others that aren't so obvious, such as some common internal discomforts throughout the body.

Using the holistic approach is going to help you to build a good foundation for helping your baby to stay healthy. A physical activity program designed for your personal situation can work in concert with eating a diet that is healthy and full of great nutrients, and can make all the difference in how well your baby grows and how good you feel during the whole pregnancy.

A holistic approach brings a wider range of tools and options to support you through your pregnancy. For example, acupuncture and massage, as long as they are done with someone certified for pregnancy, can help to provide some comfort during this time and will lower your risk of developing some of the more undesirable side effects that show up in some pregnancies. If you are having a lot of trouble during your pregnancy, consider using the holistic approach to find ways to make it a little better.

### Emotional Benefits

Having a baby is a very emotional time. While most people expect you to always be happy and excited about your baby, it can be a little bit difficult. Sure, you are excited to bring in a new life into the world and can't wait to meet your newborn, but there are a lot of hormones in play that are going all over the place, making it difficult to just feel happiness and joy all the time.

During pregnancy, you could feel sadness, anxiety, worry, and stress. Add on some of the discomforts that come naturally from the pregnancy, then add on the lack of sleep that comes towards the end of your pregnancy and the beginning of your time as a parent, and you will find that being happy all of the time is pretty much impossible.

When you use the holistic approach, you are going to learn how to acknowledge these emotions, realizing that they are a natural part of your pregnancy. You will be able to work on finding the right strategies to reduce the stress levels and cope in a healthy way with all the surging emotions as they come up.

When you learn how to cope with stress, you will be able to handle your emotions and feel more in control. You will have more peace of mind and reduce many of the bad effects that high stress can have on your physical health. When you reduce stress, you will decrease your blood pressure and heart rate, have improved digestion, reduce muscle tension, and enhance your ability to deal with the discomfort and pain of pregnancy.

The first thing that you should work on is finding the best techniques that work for you to reduce your levels of stress. There are many options, but you may find one that you like over the others. Some options that work well include yoga, self-hypnosis, meditation, guided imagery, and breath-work.

There may be classes or teachers in your area who can help you learn how to make this work during your pregnancy.

After you have learned which technique you like the most, you should work to gain more knowledge. The more you know about your body and how it works both normally, and with differences that occur during pregnancy, the easier it is to deal with some of the stress that comes up during this time.

Being in charge during this time is important not only for your stress levels, but also for the growth and development of your new baby. You need to gain the right knowledge to ensure that you are picking out the right healthcare provider who will support you, listen to you, and work with you on a holistic approach. You need the knowledge to choose which stress-relieving techniques are going to work the best for you. Without the proper tools at your disposal, it can become problematic to feel confident as you take care of yourself during pregnancy.

### Spiritual Benefits

Not only is pregnancy a time when you are going to see changes in your physical and emotional well-being, but it is also a time when some of your spiritual perspectives may change. Many people feel that they grow spiritually when they are pregnant. Growing a new life inside of you can be an intense experience. Then, after marveling at the miracle of birth and becoming a mother, you may find your spiritual connection and awareness becoming stronger in the process.

In addition, any spiritual values, and beliefs that you had before are going to come into play even stronger now that you are pregnant and deciding for two. Some people don't like the idea of using medications during labor or going into a hospital for their birth. During pregnancy, you are going to find out how strong your beliefs are, and they will shape a lot of the decisions that you make during your pregnancy.

During your pregnancy, you should take some time to reflect on the experience. Yes, this may seem a bit difficult with all of the other things that are going on in your life, but take just a few minutes each day to reflect and ponder on your experience and how you feel deep inside during your pregnancy. Ask yourself how you can go even deeper into what you are feeling and find out what is the root of the experience, it may lead you to something greater which will affect you in the long term. Take time to practice meditation, or prayer as part of your reflection time.

Some people find that starting a journal right at the beginning of your pregnancy can be very helpful. As you progress through the pregnancy, you are going to find that it is helpful for relieving stress, and it can help you to understand more fully what it means to be a mother. Plus, it could be a nice keepsake to provide to your baby when they are older and going through a pregnancy of their own.

There are so many aspects of your life that are going to be influenced during your pregnancy. Your body is going to go through a ton of physical changes that others can see, and for some, the idea of getting that pre-pregnancy body back will seem impossible. You will feel a wide range of emotions and fears that are hard to deal with, even though everyone expects you to be happy all the time. You may also spend quite a bit of time reflecting on your current and changing beliefs and learning how they are going to influence your pregnancy.

Learning to embrace all these aspects of your health is important in ensuring that you have a healthy pregnancy. The holistic approach looks at each one of these to help you make the right decisions for both you and your unborn child. Proponents believe it to be a superior method and one that provides a more natural and organic entry into the world for your baby, as well as a warmer and more supportive pregnancy and childbirth experience for you.

# Chapter 9: Frequently Asked Questions During Pregnancy

### 1. How do I know if I am ready to get pregnant?

Thinking about if you are ready or not is a big step. When you are properly prepared, then you will be less stressed about what could or could not happen. Before you get pregnant, it is best that you got to your OB/GYN and get a checkup as well as ask any questions that you may have about childbirth and being pregnant. During this checkup, your doctor will switch you off any medications that you may be on that could harm your fetus when you become pregnant. Moreover, they will also give you the information you need when it comes to folic acid, prenatal vitamins, and everything that you need to have or know about in order to prepare your body for conception.

### 2. How do I know when is the right time for me to get pregnant?

The best time for you to get pregnant is when you are ovulating. Ovulation happens typically fourteen days before your next period is set to start (if you are on a regular schedule. This can be difficult to track if your periods are not regular). Most cycles last twenty-four to thirty days and you will begin to ovulate somewhere between day ten and day sixteen.

### 3. What are the pros and cons of getting pregnant?

Everyone looks at pregnancy differently, so there are going to be different pros and cons for every woman depending on how they look at being pregnant.

A few cons that are quite common amongst mothers are:

• The decisions that you must make with regards to getting prenatal screenings, what you are going to do with the results, so on and so forth.

• The lack of alcohol. You are not supposed to drink while you are pregnant. Even though some doctors will tell you that it is okay for you to have a glass or two in moderation, there are others who will tell you to stay away from it completely. It is up to you on whether you heed their warning.

• How pregnancy is going to affect your body. Yes, your body is going to change because you are having a child that is growing in your womb thus making not only your abdomen extend as they get bigger, but changing things such as how your breasts appear and things like that.

• Mood swings and lack of sleep. Thanks to the number of hormones that are flooding your system, you may find that you are more irritable at times than others and that you are having problems sleeping when your baby gets here.

Some pros are:

• Bigger breasts. As you go through your pregnancy, your breasts are going to grow large due to the milk that is being produced in preparation for the breastfeeding process.

• Being spoiled with love and care. Many women experience that their partners, their friends, and their families tend to spoil them when they find out that they are pregnant because everyone is excited about the baby!

• Your hair and nails are going to grow faster thanks to all those hormones (they are not all bad, they just tend to get a little bit irritating when it comes to certain aspects of your pregnancy).

## 4. What foods do I avoid during pregnancy?

It is suggested that you need to stay away from:

• Fish that contains a lot of mercury. Having large amounts of mercury in your system can end up damaging a developing brain.

• You should also stay away from any unpasteurized soft cheeses such as brie, feta, gorgonzola, etc.

• Raw fish such as sushi.

• Cold ready to eat meals like hot dogs or lunch meat because of the listeria that the meat can contain.

• Unpasteurized milk (which is also a source of listeria).

• Alcohol because it can interfere with the development of your fetus and even lead to fetal alcohol syndrome.

• Uncooked or cured eggs and meats such as prosciutto, or runny eggs.

• Caffeine however it is okay when you take it in moderate amounts.

## 5. What foods should I eat while I am pregnant?

Above all, you need to follow a healthy diet and your body

needs extra vitamins and minerals. Whatever anybody may tell you, you do not need to 'eat for two'. It is advised that you eat an extra 350 to 500 calories (1470 to 2090 kilojoules) during the 2nd and 3rd trimesters. If your diet is lacking, it may affect the baby's growth.

Unhealthy eating habits and gaining excess weight can put you at a greater danger of gestational diabetes, or birth difficulties. Things such as leafy greens, vegetables, fruits, whole grain bread and cereals are going to be the best option, while you are pregnant. You also need to consume food that contains protein and calcium, such as low-fat yogurts, broccoli, eggs, salmon. When it comes to meat, please refer to the portion on what not to eat, but above all make sure the meat is cooked thoroughly!

### 6. Does it matter if I miss a day of my pregnancy vitamins?

Prenatal vitamins are important in helping to bridge the gap in any of the nutrients that you may be missing in your diet. However, if you happen to miss a day or two of your prenatal vitamins, you are not going to find that anything is going to happen to you or your baby. There are some women who never take prenatal vitamins when they are pregnant.

### 7. What should I do if I become constipated during pregnancy?

Constipation is something that many pregnant women

complain about. This is not too uncommon for women at some point in their pregnancy. With all the progesterone in your system, you are going to realize that your muscles are smoothed out and relaxed, and this also affects the digestive tract.

Due to all the progesterone, your food is going to pass through your digestive system slower. Not only that but taking iron supplements in high doses is going to cause you to have constipation.

### To combat constipation, you can:

☐ Drink plenty of water

Your urine should look clear. One glass of juice a day will help as well, most particularly prune juice to help regulate your digestive system. There have been reports that drinking some sort of warm liquid after you get up will also help to keep you from being constipated.

☐ Eat foods that are high in fiber

This should be things such as whole-grain bread and cereals along with brown rice, beans, and fresh vegetables and fruits. You can also include a tablespoon or two of unprocessed wheat bran with your breakfast along with a glass of water to help you get things moving.

☐ Look at your prenatal vitamins

If they contain a high amount of iron, then ask your healthcare provider about switching to a different prenatal that does not have so much iron in it. The only reason that you need a lot of iron is because you are anemic and are needing to increase your iron intake.

☐ Exercise regularly

Doing light exercises such as swimming, yoga, riding a stationary bike, or even walking can help you to ease the pain of constipation and leave you not only feeling better, but feeling healthier.

☐ After you eat, use the bathroom.

Your body knows when you need to get rid of the waste in it; so, listen to it. Do not put off going to the bathroom once you feel the need to. Doing this can cause problems later.

If all else fails, talk to your doctor about prescribing you something that can help or about adding an over the counter fiber supplement or even stool softener to your daily routine.

The only time that you should begin to worry about your constipation is if there are other symptoms with it such as, abdominal pain, you are passing mucus or blood, or you are having constipation and then diarrhea alternating. At this point in time, you need to get in contact with your doctor or other health care provider as it may be a different issue that is causing this.

While you are going to the bathroom, try not to strain. If you strain you can end up causing hemorrhoids or even cause them to worsen if you already have them. This is caused by the swelling of the veins in your rectal area.

Hemorrhoids are painful and uncomfortable but will end up going away when you give birth to your baby. If you find that the pain is too severe or you are having bleeding from your rectal, you need to call your health care provider to see if there is a more serious issue going on.

## 8. What exercises can I do while I am pregnant?

While you are pregnant, you can do activities such as swimming, walking, a stationary bike, low impact aerobics, a step machine, and even an elliptical machine. You can also do things such as tennis, racquetball, and jogging.

However, you need to be careful and talk to your health care provider if you are unsure if you should be doing the activity.

## 9. What are my exercise limitations while I am pregnant?

Most exercises you are going to be able to do and you are probably going to slow down and change your routines as your abdomen gets bigger. However, you are going to want to avoid things that are going to give you a higher risk of falling or any kind of abdominal injury.

Along with those, you are going to want to avoid any high-altitude sports.

### 10. Can I have sex while I am pregnant?

Yes!

If your partner fears having intercourse with you while you are pregnant. Reassure him that he is not going to hurt you or the baby. If he is still unsure about it, then talk to your doctor about ways that you can help calm his fears so you can get back to doing what you want to do.

### 11. What is first trimester screening?

This is a test that is done early in your pregnancy to offer some information about the chromosomal risks for things such as Down syndrome. Testing is done by either a blood test or an ultrasound exam.

### 12. What do I do with my first trimester screening results?

Your results are going to tell you if your baby is at risk for Down syndrome. This test does not mean that your child will have Down syndrome, it only tells you the risk of carrying a baby with this genetic condition.

## 13. What symptoms are normal while I am pregnant?

There are different symptoms that you will experience while you are pregnant, however, some of the symptoms you may experience are:

- Swelling and bloating,
- Acne,
- Cramping,
- Changes in your sleep pattern,
- Sensitivities

## 14. Is it normal to have extra discharge while pregnant?

Yes. Not only are your hormones sky-rocketing due to your baby, you also have extra blood flow going to your pelvis. There is a high possibility that you are going to notice an increase in discharge as you go through your pregnancy.

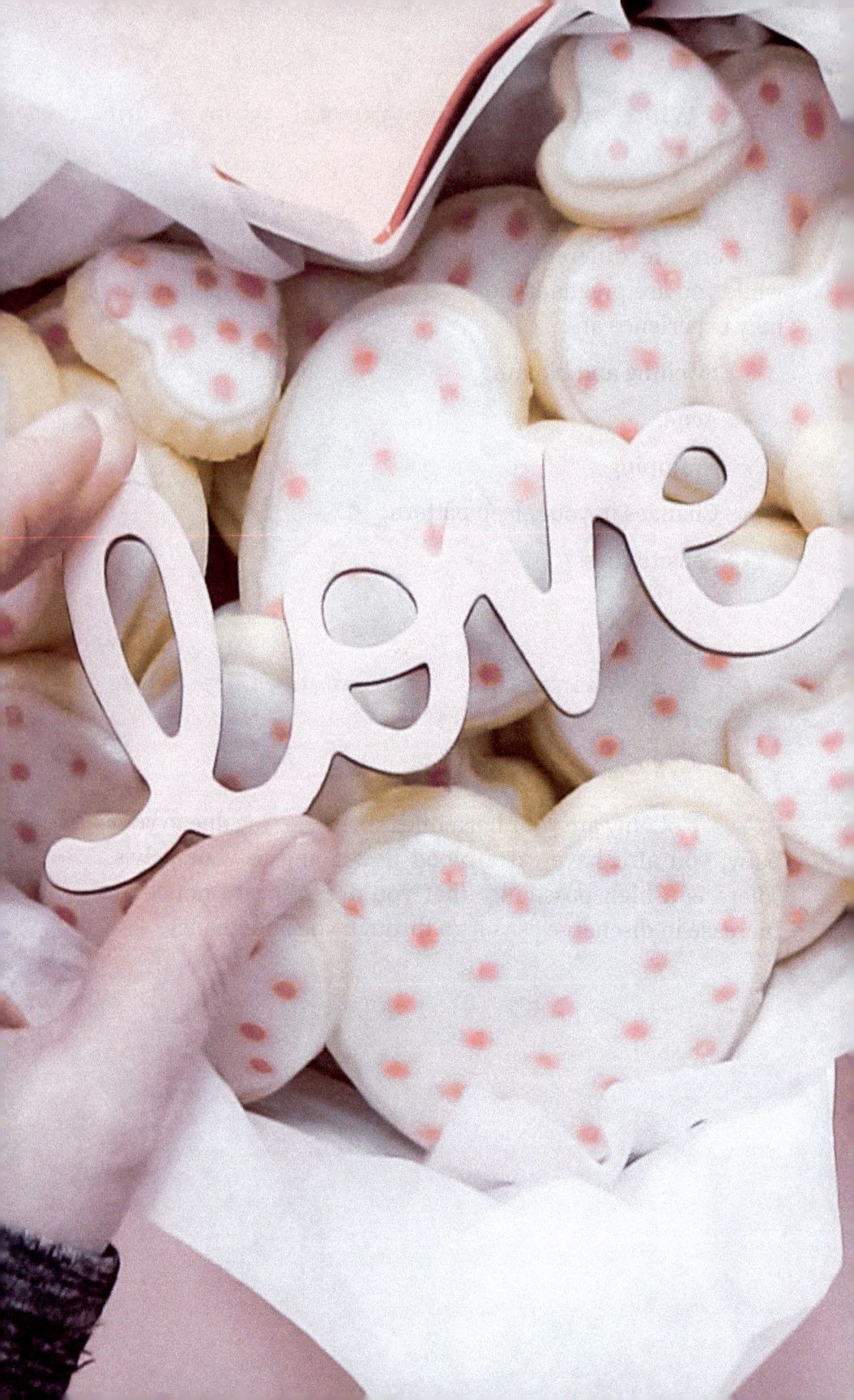

# Part 3: The Third Trimester: Accepting and Preparing for a Significant Change to Your Identity

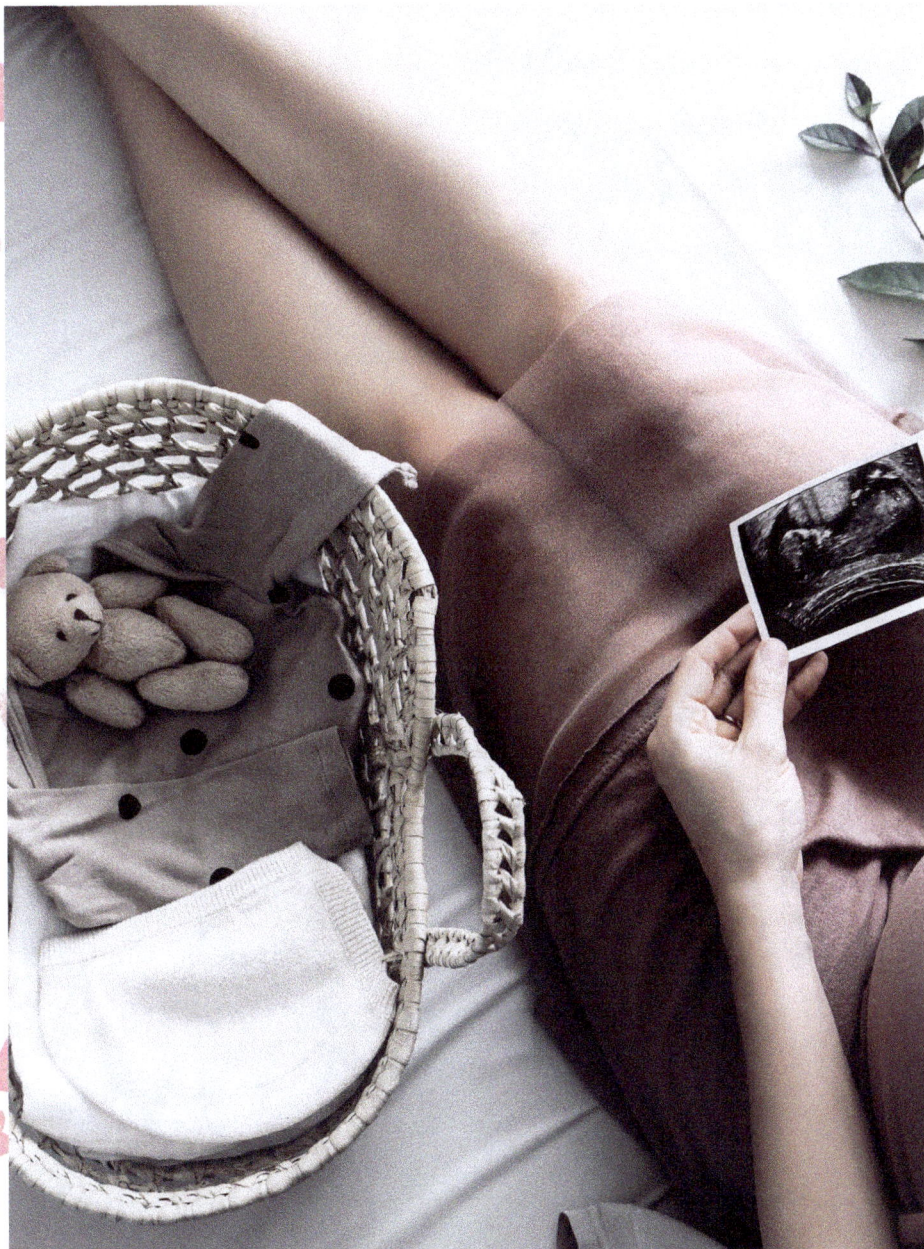

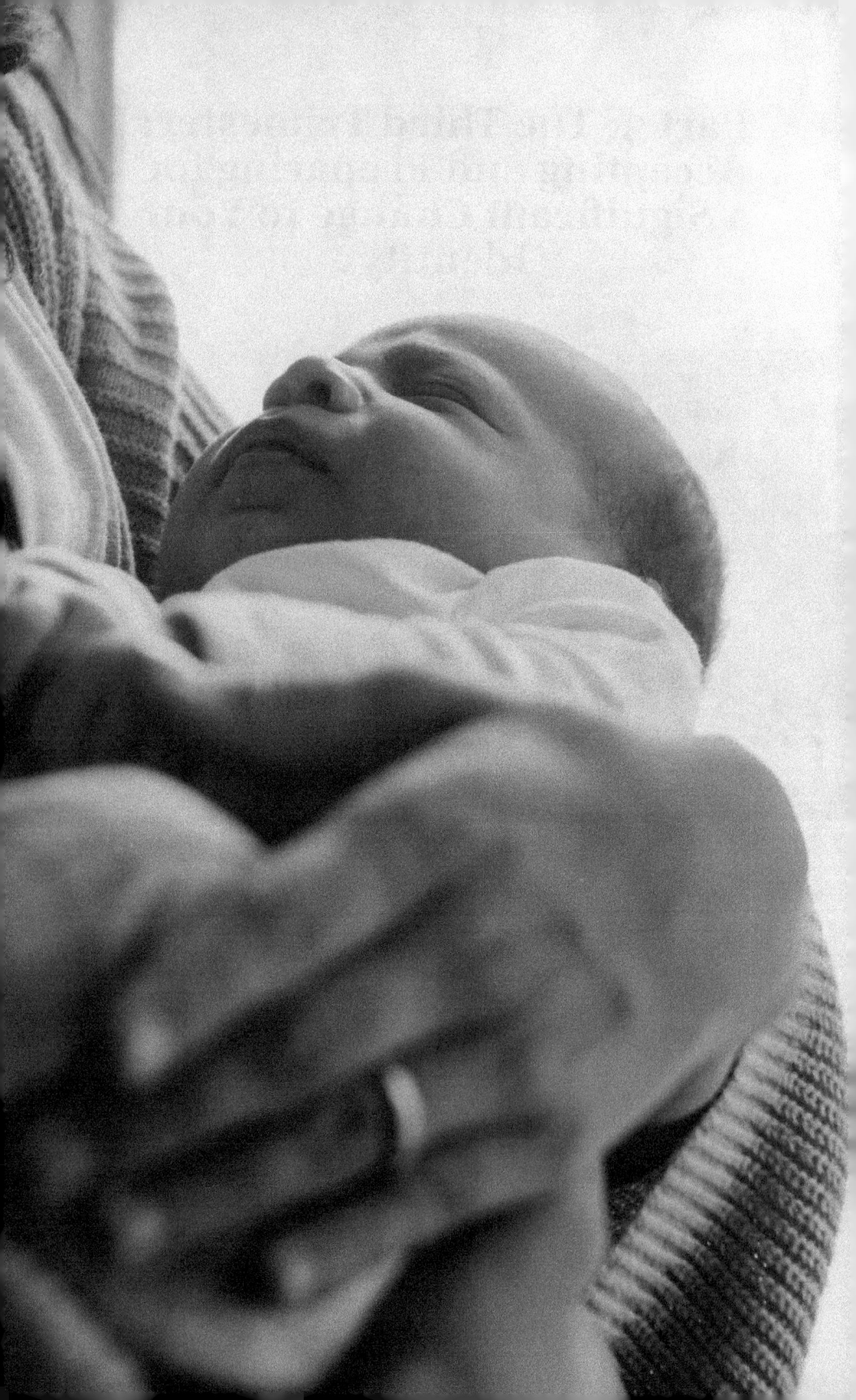

# Chapter 10: How to Become A Mother Without Losing Yourself?

Everything flows from you, as the mother, so you need to take care of yourself to be an effective mother and nurture your exciting relationships. Motherhood comes with many pressures, so the pressure must not come from yourself. You play a major role in the process as mothers usually feel more attached to their children since they developed inside of their wombs. This is a time to focus on yourself as opposed to your partner or child. I want you to say out loud that you matter and that you are going to put yourself first. It's mommy time.

Scheduling time for yourself can seem extremely difficult in the early days as you are trying to balance your schedule. Your priorities are just trying to make sure that your child is well taken care of. This is not an incorrect approach because your child should come first but I want you to also think of yourself. In the early days, you might be shocked to find that you haven't washed your hair in a week or that you've been wearing the same sweatpants for a full week. Your appearance is the last thing you'll think about or even prioritize. I need you to take some time for your appearance even if it's just a few minutes a day to brush your hair. It might sound silly but a few minutes of just brushing your hair and preparing for the day will impact your outlook of the day. You'll be in a better headspace so you will be able to take better care of your child. You need to prioritize self-care to be successful. There are other small things that you can do to lift your spirits, like making your bath time more enjoyable. You might not have a full hour to soak in the tub but just by playing some light music or lighting a few candles for a 20-minute soak you can feel more energized. A helpful tip is to schedule your baths around your child's naptime. This allows you to take care of yourself without having to wonder about what's happening with your baby. If you keep the baby monitor near you during this time, you can keep an eye on your child. When your child begins to have a more consistent sleep schedule it will become much easier for you to plan moments for yourself.

Gratitude will play a huge role in this period because you need to remind yourself of how precious every day is. Your child is growing and developing in front of you daily. It can be easy to take this for granted because of increased stress levels of fatigue but you need to remind yourself to be grateful. You can start your morning or finish off your day with a gratitude check by writing down what moment you are grateful for. This can be your child's laughter, a show you enjoyed watching, or even just that you got through the day. A gratitude journal is a great way to look back at what you've been through and the moments that you might have forgotten about. It allows you to recognize how far you and your baby have come. You will experience a different kind of fulfillment from your child that will change your outlook on life.

It's important to allow yourself room to grow and develop while still not completely altering your being. If you were a happy person before, then there's no reason why you shouldn't be that now. The aim is not to lose yourself during this transition, but just allowing your personality to develop with you. Gratitude allows you to enjoy the motherhood journey.

A great way to make time for yourself and all the changes that you have experienced is to give yourself a mommy makeover. Your fashion choices will need to be adjusted a little to fit your new body. Your style does not need to change, but you can buy yourself more comfortable alternatives. If you loved constantly wearing jeans that might not be the most comfortable idea straight after giving birth. You can still feel dressed up by switching your jeans for a stylish pair of jeggings. You don't have to say goodbye to your favorite summer dresses, you can just try different styles and cuts to suit your body. You can still be fashionable even as a mother. There has always been this stereotype that mothers must look a certain way or can't wear certain styles. All these ideas are outdated and there is a consensus that it's perfectly fine for moms to be considered sexy or attractive. Your clothing choices can positively impact how you feel about yourself. Once you have your clothes right then a new hairstyle might be in order. Getting a haircut or coloring your hair is a great way to step out of your comfort zone and introduce yourself as a mom. A haircut that doesn't require a lot of maintenance is a great move for a new mom. We all know that a trip to the hairdresser feels like a form of therapy for many of us, so make time to go. If you can arrange for your hairdresser to do a home visit that's a great alternative for moms who are not ready to leave the house yet, although a change of scenery is highly recommended. A trip to a day spa or your local manicurist is a fun short trip that can-do wonders for your confidence levels.

Try treating yourself with a manicure or pedicure occasionally. Just be sure to get a nail shape and length that doesn't impact how you function daily. Claw shaped nails might have been a good idea before you had your baby but now, they are probably just going to unintentionally scratch your baby. The main way not to lose yourself in this phase is by finding the time to do the things that you enjoy and finding new hobbies. If you love reading, then try reading a part a day of a book you love. The point isn't to feel obligated or stressed out about finding windows to pamper yourself, but it's about enjoying this time.

You need to take ownership of your body after pregnancy. The process was affected by your decisions, but you could not completely control the outcome. Your body became a home for a whole other person and once that person moved out, they left a few markers of their presence. It can be hard for you to come to terms with the changes regardless of how excited you are to have a child. You need to be comfortable in your skin, as this can negatively affect your relationship if you do not. This comfort leads to confidence in yourself. Confidence will always be a desirable quality in anyone and more specifically in a first-time mother who trusts in her abilities. Trust me, your partner will be totally attracted to this confidence and assertiveness that you have. A great way to regain your confidence is to spoil yourself with new lingerie. You will be grateful for the new pieces and the confidence that it gives you. Lingerie is another great way to get closer to your partner post-pregnancy. It allows you to be more comfortable with your body and enjoy your new body. Sleep plays a major role in your outlook on life because it impacts how much time to rest your body is getting. Sleep deprivation is very harmful to your mental health and your general physical health. When you are sleep deprived, you are less alert and more likely to intentionally cause harm to yourself or others. Getting enough sleep is an act of self-care because it directly affects your well-being. If you find that you aren't getting enough sleep, then talk to the support system around you about helping out with your child during the day so you can rest for a few hours, or take turns with your partner for nightly feedings.

Self-care includes knowing when to ask those around you for help regardless of what that help is. This could be asking for assistance with your laundry, cooking or just tidying up around your home. You'd be surprised at how quickly your home can feel like a complete mess after a few days of not doing dishes. We live in an age where there is a phone application for anything you can think of. Be sure to use this to your advantage by making your life easier and hiring cleaning services, beauty appointments or grocery deliveries. The idea of hiring someone else to do your household tasks through an application might seem foreign at first but it's a great way to save yourself time. These services are relatively affordable and very easy to book. A great tool you can add to your life is monthly subscription services that can offer you a variety of goods. They range from beauty tools, wine subscriptions, food deliveries, children's' products or even clothing. The knowledge that once a month there is something specifically delivered for you is a great way to pamper yourself. I love subscription services because whenever I receive a package it always feels like a gift to myself. This is especially true for subscription services that don't specify what is in their boxes. You will know the general theme but not the specific item. It's a great way to discover new products and services. The wine subscriptions are great for moms who want to host people in their homes. A book club is a great way to socialize with other people who have a similar schedule to you.

Your identity as a mother isn't an overnight switch, which is why it's important to decide what you want it to be. If it's a conscious decision, then you can control your outlook. It helps if you take a moment and take a few moments out of your day to just take stock of how you have adjusted to motherhood; you will be able to see whether or not you are where you want to be. Your situation will not be the same as anyone else's, so it's important to identify your path. Are you a stay at home mom, a working mom, or a bit of both? This helps you stay accountable and make time for all the things you want to do. If you want to be a stay at home mom, then you can plan your days around your daily goals and tasks. If you want to stay at home while still making time for your work, then you need to balance out your schedule to suit your needs. It's about finding what works for you and your family. Your identity is who you were before you were a mother and who you want to be after becoming a mother. Your life can seem to center around your child's needs and wants but you need to not only live for your child but yourself as well. New moms often feel lost because their child's schedule takes precedence above their own. You might feel like all your freedoms have been stripped away but they haven't, you just need to rebalance your mind and change your outlook.

# Chapter 11: Financial Planning for Parenthood and its Impact on Your Partnership

## *The High Cost of Having A Baby*

If you have substantial or full insurance coverage for your prenatal care and delivery expenses, you can breathe a sigh of relief. According to an Agency for Healthcare Research and Quality report released in 2010, average hospital charges for delivering a baby in 2008 were $3,400 for an uncomplicated delivery and $5,700 for an uncomplicated cesarean section. The average cost climbs to $9,400 for a vaginal delivery with an operating procedure. And prenatal care adds another several thousand to the bill; however, studies show that such expenses are more than offset by improved outcomes for both mother and child.

## Insurance Issues

Review your insurance plan so that you are clear on the extent and nature of your coverage for both prenatal care and labor and delivery. If you have questions, call your insurance company, or speak to the benefits coordinator at your workplace.

Keep on top of insurance problems. As any physician's or hospital's billing department can tell you, insurance companies do occasionally lose and mishandle claims. Whenever you call either your provider's billing department or the insurance company, take notes summarizing the conversation, including a date to follow up, and the name of the person you speak with. If you're trying to unravel a knotty insurance issue, being able to track it with someone who is familiar with your case will save you time and aggravation. And if you aren't getting action, it helps to document exactly who has dropped the ball as you move up the chain of command. Follow up with letters and request written documentation of any actions taken over the phone so that you have a paper trail as well.

## Payment Options

If you have a large deductible to pay out of pocket or are responsible for a hefty percentage of your physician's bill, don't panic. Work with your provider's office to negotiate a realistic payment schedule. Contact the business office of the hospital or birthing center where you will deliver for registration information and details on their billing terms. Some providers and hospitals may have maternity assistance programs, including sliding fee scales and prepayment discounts.

### Ways to Save

According to the U.S. Census Bureau estimates, 16.7 percent of all Americans were without health insurance in 2009. There are public aid programs available if you are uninsured and unable to meet the financial obligations of prenatal care and childbirth.

Medicaid is a state-run public assistance program that provides medical care to low-income families at little to no cost. For information on qualifying standards, see the federal Centers for Medicare and Medicaid Services' website at www.cms.gov or call your state social services department.

The Special Supplemental Nutrition Program for Women,

Infants, and Children (WIC) is a federally funded, state-administered program targeted to nutritionally at-risk women (both pregnant and postpartum) and children up to age 5. WIC provides food vouchers to those who meet qualifying guidelines and have a yearly gross household income that does not surpass 185 percent of the federal poverty level ($41,348 for a family of four in the forty-eight contiguous states in 2011; slightly higher in Alaska and Hawaii).

The Children's Health Insurance Program (CHIP) is a federal program that covers infants and children in families that are financially strained but earn income levels too high to qualify for Medicaid. If you're concerned about insurance coverage for your newborn, call 1-877-KIDS-NOW or visit www.insurekidsnow.gov for more details.

There may be other financial assistance available in your area. Contact your area social services agency for more details.

### Bargain Hunters

Even if you've never been one to clip coupons, the expense of keeping baby in diapers and other essentials is a strong incentive to start looking for savings. Next time you're at the doctor's office, look around the waiting room for product offers. Many new-parent clubs have cropped up, supported by formula makers, diaper manufacturers, and other baby product companies, and they often recruit members right there at the source.

Some kid-focused retailers also have coupon clubs. Sign up if you'd like to receive free product samples and coupons. One caveat: putting your name on their mailing lists may open you up to a deluge of junk mail from so-called "valued partners." Check out the form you sign for its printed privacy policy if this is a concern; it may offer you an opportunity to opt out of such mailings.

There are several free magazines on the market geared specifically for new parents and moms-to-be, again often available right at your provider's office. Be aware that because the publishers make their money from advertisers rather than from subscribers, these publications are typically laden with product ads. However, they still have lots of useful new parenting information and an abundance of coupons and free offers.

Check your local library for other community or regional parenting publications that can point you toward useful family resources and, again, those handy coupons.

Although breast milk is the least expensive way to feed your baby (along with its many other extraordinary health benefits), if you are planning on bottle-feeding, freebies abound. The formula is expensive, and the baby will eventually be putting away about 30 ounces a day (900 ounces per month). Acquiring a loyal customer through free samples and other incentives makes good business sense to formula manufacturers, who are big on the new-parent clubs. They also provide a steady stream of samples to prenatal care providers and pediatricians. If you don't see samples or aren't offered any, ask your provider.

Finally, if you deliver in a hospital, make sure you get what you pay for. Chances are you'll be billed for all the items you and your newborn use—including the pacifier, nasal aspirator, sanitary napkins, alcohol swabs, open bags of diapers and wipe cloths, and even the little plastic comb for baby's hair (whether the baby has any or not). Take these with you when you leave! Ask the nurse what is fair game. Often the hospital staff can send you home with even more free product samples than you will find in your hospital room.

## Financial Planning for a Bigger Family

Clueless about baby care costs? Take a reconnaissance mission to the grocery store to gather prices on diapers, wipes, and other essentials. If you're considering day care or an in-home babysitter, now is also a good time to get information and monthly cost estimates. As usual, other parents are an excellent source of tips and leads to the best resources in your area.

Don't forget to factor in pediatric care and additional health insurance premiums on your bottom line. If you belong to an HMO or other managed-care health plan, it's probable that well-baby visits are covered at 100 percent or with a minimal copay. You may want to review your health insurance options now so that when the baby comes you can enroll her in the most appropriate and cost-effective program.

## Setting Savings Goals

Now that you've figured out what you'll be spending on baby care, of what practical use is this? Lay out your current spending habits, including basic monthly bills like utilities and housing, debts that can be downsized (for example, credit cards and car payments), transportation costs, food and household goods, health-care, and discretionary/disposable income. Accounting for everything in black and white will give you a much clearer picture of where you're spending and the size of any gap between income and expenses. This can also help you figure out big-picture questions like whether you have the financial means to switch to a part-time schedule at work.

When it comes time to balance your home budget, be realistic in your planning and prudent when you eliminate discretionary purchases; brown-bagging it to work each and every day for the next 3 years is a noble goal, but a weekly or biweekly meal out with colleagues could pay off in other ways. Give yourself a little breathing room for unforeseen emergency expenses like an appliance meltdown or car repairs. A little scrimping here, one less latte a week there, and you'll find budgeting easier than you thought.

Some parents find it daunting to consider long-term expenses, like college, when the costs and responsibilities of child rearing itself seem so overwhelming. Just remember that early planning can net big returns over time. If you start saving just $50 a month in a savings account or other interest-bearing investment at a 5 percent interest rate when your child is born, you will have $16,026 by the time your child is ready to start college. If you don't know an IRA from the NRA, you might want to sit down with a financial advisor to discuss college savings options. She might also be able to assist you in re-evaluating your life insurance needs, something else that should be done periodically as your family grows.

### Lifestyle Changes, Or Stating the Obvious

Your baby's arrival will transform just about everything you think, say, and do. This sea change is usually most evident with first-time parents, who up until now have been enjoying the child-free pursuits of quiet dinners, R-rated movies, and even the occasional wild night out with the girls or boys. Even those moms and dads who are expecting a second or subsequent child will have big adjustments ahead with new challenges like siblinghood and advanced parental multitasking (for example, encouraging one child to use his napkin while preventing the other from eating hers). Don't look at it as an end but rather as a new and infinitely more rewarding part of your life. You will even find some family pastimes you have never considered before.

## Sharing Pregnancy with the Dad-to-Be

With the big focus on mom and her growing belly, it's easy for dads to get overlooked in the pregnancy drama. Remind your significant other that you're in this together. If he isn't quite sure of his role in this new adventure yet, he could be looking to you for cues. Encourage him to join you at prenatal checkups as well as share pregnancy education and experiences like the first kicks. You should also try to pencil in some special couple time to talk to baby, contemplate names, and share your hopes and dreams about your family's future.

## From Two to Three

The new person in your life has already started competing for your attention, changing your eating, and sleeping patterns, and perhaps slowing down your pace. Unexpected emotions may surface between you and your significant other as your pregnancy progresses. He may feel pangs of jealousy at the loss of your couple hood and your focus on the baby. On the flip side, you may be feeling as if you're playing second fiddle to your future child as the prospective father questions the safety of every move you make. Such growing pains are normal. Try to talk about your feelings and approach parenting (even now) as a team effort.

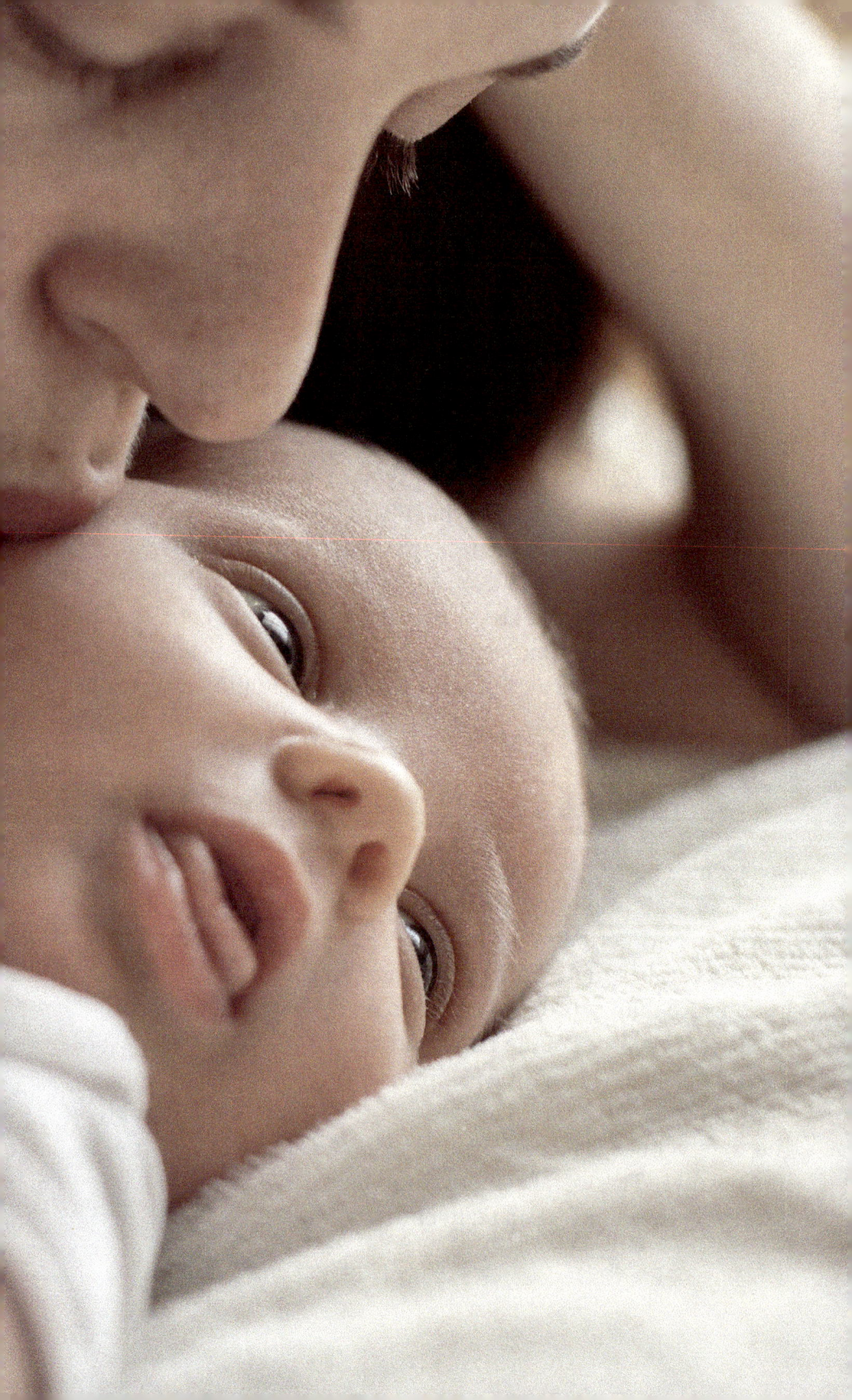

# Chapter 12: Labor and Delivery: Facing One of Life's Most Intense Experiences

S o, it's the real deal. You are in labor. The contractions are getting stronger and the baby is on the way. Some woman has a long labor and some woman have a quick labor. Normally, for first time moms, labor is going to be longer than shorter. You may want visitors to come and see you and you may not. Remember it is up to you!

If you want privacy, then utilize your nurse to kick everybody out! Your partner will be there, and they are there for you! Squeeze their hand as hard as you need to! They can take it. Heck, you're the one in labor! When contractions get around four minutes apart you can get your epidural. Now is not the time to be a hero. If you need the drugs, then you get the drugs! You will still feel the pressure and you will still feel your baby born. It will just remove the pain out of the equation.

Truth time. Labor can be embarrassing at times. You are going to get checked down below by more than one person. The birth of your child is no time to be shy. If at any time you want the nurse to check your progress than speak up and ask. Your nurse may act like she knows more about your body, but you are the smartest when it comes to your body. You will push when you are 100% effaced and ten centimeters dilated. When it is time to push the stirrups come out and the lights go on. There is going to be a flurry of activity and a lot of medical personnel coming in. This is the time to kick out any guests you don't want there for the big reveal.

When you are pushing you will push for ten seconds and then take a break and push again. You only push during contractions. The contractions can be very close together at this point and so you may feel as though you are continually pushing. Pushing can be done in minutes or in hours. There is really no way to tell. You can do it! You are a superwoman! For nine months you have carried a child inside your body, and you deserve to meet her. Ice chips can help during labor. Ask your partner to rub the small of your back, if you don't mind being touched, and it will help alleviate some of the discomforts. When you are pushing the nurse is going to ask you to bear down. You basically are pushing all your energy down near your rectum. Truth time. There is a very good chance that you will have a bowel movement on the table. It can be embarrassing but just let it go and don't worry about it. Labor and delivery nurses are completely used to it and will just wipe it up and go without a second thought.

There is a chance you could need to have a C-section. Possibly you have a medical condition that requires this. The baby may be a breach (which means he is turned the wrong way) and the doctor is unable to turn her. The baby's heartbeat may be going too fast or too slow or labor is not progressing, and the doctor decides that the baby will be better off being born by C-section. Maybe you were really wanting to experience the delivery. It can be hard to adjust. However, you want what is best for your baby and it will be all right.

You most likely will have the option to watch the birth in the mirror. If you do not want to watch that is ok! Either decision is perfectly natural and ok. You may also find that you are so absorbed in giving birth that you forget to look! If you want pictures or videos of the birth that is your decision and you do need to decide this with your partner before you get to the hospital. All right, here it is! Last push. You are going to feel a strange sliding sensation and then feel the baby enter the world.

Hello Baby! The staff will lie that baby right down on you. Oh yeah, you are probably bawling your eyes out. No matter what this beautiful life looks life; this child is the most beautiful thing you have ever seen. You will love his little fingers and her cute little face. You get to say "hello baby" to your child for the first time. You will hear the baby cry for the first time. All these things are truly amazing, and you will never forget them. Take a moment and soak it all in. You are a mommy!

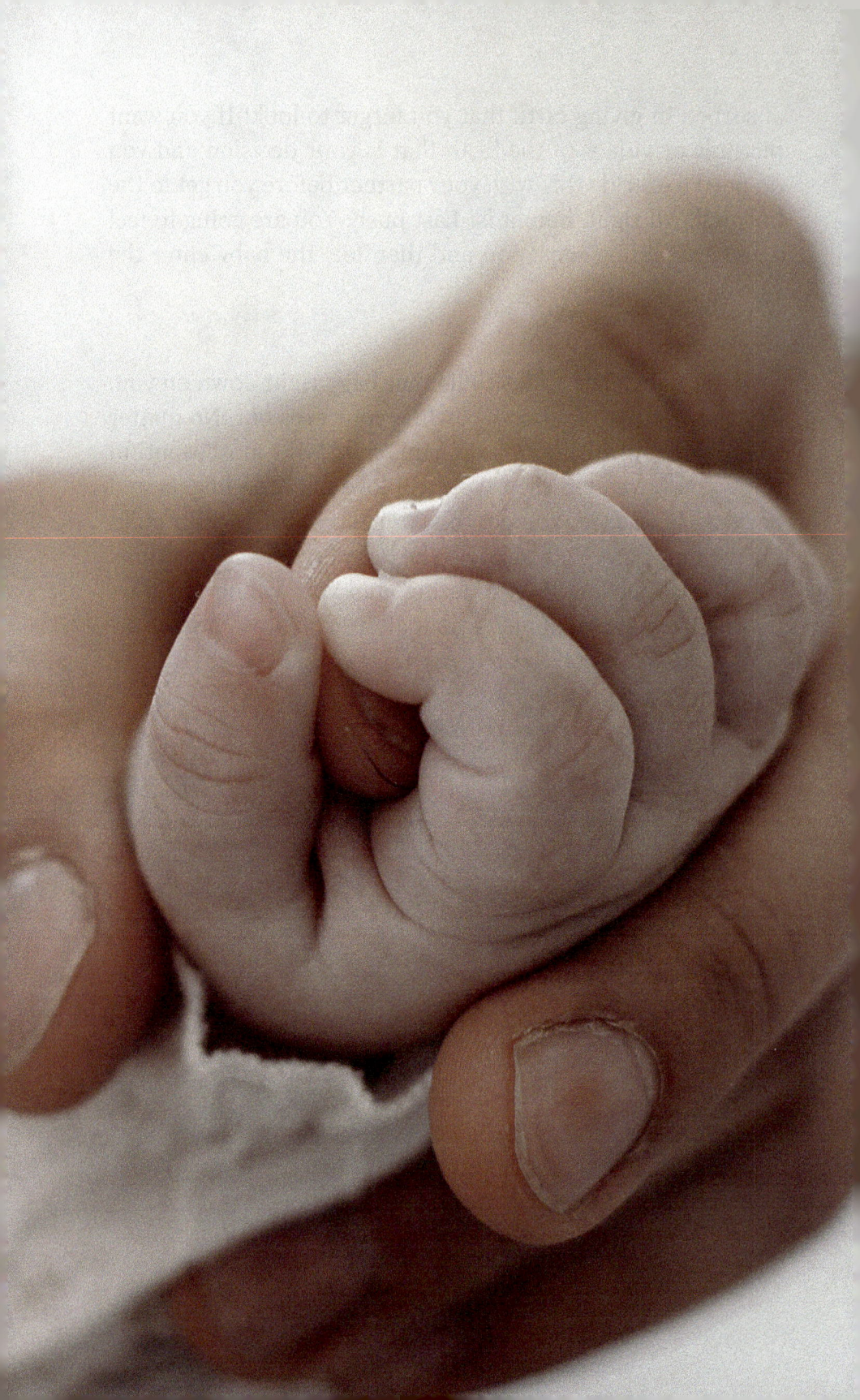

# Part 4: Uncomfortable Questions

### *Will I Poop in the Delivery Room?*

Many patients ask about the solid discharge during the labor process. This is very common, and there is nothing to be ashamed of. The attendant will take care of any poop that occurs during the pregnancy. You and your partner do not have to worry about this as it is perfectly normal.

- What if we don't make it to the birth center in time?
- What if my baby is breech?
- What if I have back labor?

### *What if my labor stalls?*

Patients consistently ask, "How long along am I?" and we have trouble furnishing them an exact response. Pregnancy is said to last for nine months; however, that number isn't exact. From the last menstrual period, the pregnancy lasts for 40 weeks or 280 days. (You think 40 weeks is quite a while? Simply be happy you're not an elephant, which has a growth time of 22 months!) When you are pregnant, you ought to be in the pregnancy phase for at least ten months – calculating the time from when you know you are pregnant to delivering a healthy baby. On the schedule, most months contain a month in addition to a few days, so nine schedule months frequently contain near 40 weeks. Professionals talk as far as weeks when estimating gestational age since it's progressively exact and less befuddling.

### Others Can Drive You Crazy

Companions, family members, associates, outsiders, and even your partner can offer you spontaneous assessments, guidance and need to impart to your pregnancy depending on their knowledge and experience they have accumulated. They might suggest awful opinions that might make you angry such as your back looks large, you're excessively fat (or excessively meager), or you shouldn't eat anything that you're placing in your mouth.

You should understand that these individuals, have honest goals when they disclose to you how their sister's pregnancy finished severely, or about the issue a companion of a companion had. They don't understand that they're expanding your tension. Try not to focus. Attempt to grin and overlook them obligingly.

### You Will Feel Exhausted in the First Trimester

You might some feel weakness in the first trimester, this is because your body will be coming up with the changes in your body. You will also feel the urge to get additional sleep. Be it at the labor place or the transit, hence, you will always be wanting to get some rest. You need to know that this weakness will go away, and you will not feel tired in the second and third trimester. The tiredness will wear off in the 13th week, but you need to make sure you give proper rest to your body in the first three months of pregnancy. You will also feel the same tiredness when you are close to the labor process. Around week 30, the same feeling will be engulfing you for a month.

### Round Ligament Pain Really Hurts

The round tendons are in the bottom part of the body and are located between the uterus and labia. When you are pregnant, the uterus will expand, and this will cause the tendons to stretch. The pain is caused due to the stretchiness of the tendons. You will feel some pain in the crotch area between the 16 and 22 weeks of pregnancy. The pain that accompanies the stretchiness of the tendons will end, so there is no need to be worried about them. Changing the position regularly will also help in eliminating the pain. The pain will be completely gone by the 24 weeks.

### Your Belly Becomes a Hand Magnet

After your stomach projects recognizably with pregnancy, you're probably going to discover all of a sudden everybody presumes contacting it is alright — not just your companions, relatives, and the individuals you labor with, yet in addition the postal laborer, the clerk at the store, and others you've never at any point met. Few ladies value the additional consideration, many thinks that it's an intrusion of privacy. You can either smile or bear with them.

### Hemorrhoids Are a Royal Pain in the Butt

Due to the change in the shifting weights, you might feel some pain in the bottom part of the body. It is best to consult your doctor when you feel this pain. This pain will mostly be gone within fourteen days. In case you're lucky enough not to have them, understand how fortunate you are — and have compassion toward the various new moms who do have them.

### The Weight Stays On after the Baby Comes Out

When a woman gives birth to the baby and the placenta, the woman will shed some weight. The woman may also have some swelling in the hands and feet, which is completely normal. This additional water maintenance includes pounds. If you step on the scale immediately, you might be disillusioned at the number that surfaces. The expanding, for the most part, it takes about up to 14 days to leave.

Medical Clinic Pads are Relics from Your Mother's Era

At certain medical clinics, the attendants offer you sterile napkins from the 1920s — and a charming minimal, versatile belt to hang them on. In case you're a time traveler or if for some other explanation you favor this sort, fantastic. You can also bring your home pads and containers for additional support.

### Breast Engorgement Really Sucks, and Breast-encouraging Can Be a Production

When you deliver the baby, you might feel that your breasts become hard and big. The milk production also starts when the baby is delivered. We empower our patients to bosom feed because of the wellbeing of for the child; however, remember it might be more earnestly than you might suspect. Requiring some additional assistance and help is extremely regular. Luckily, most clinics have lactation masters that can assist you with draining the procedure along.

# Part 5: Mindful Preparation for Birth Plans and Birth Classes

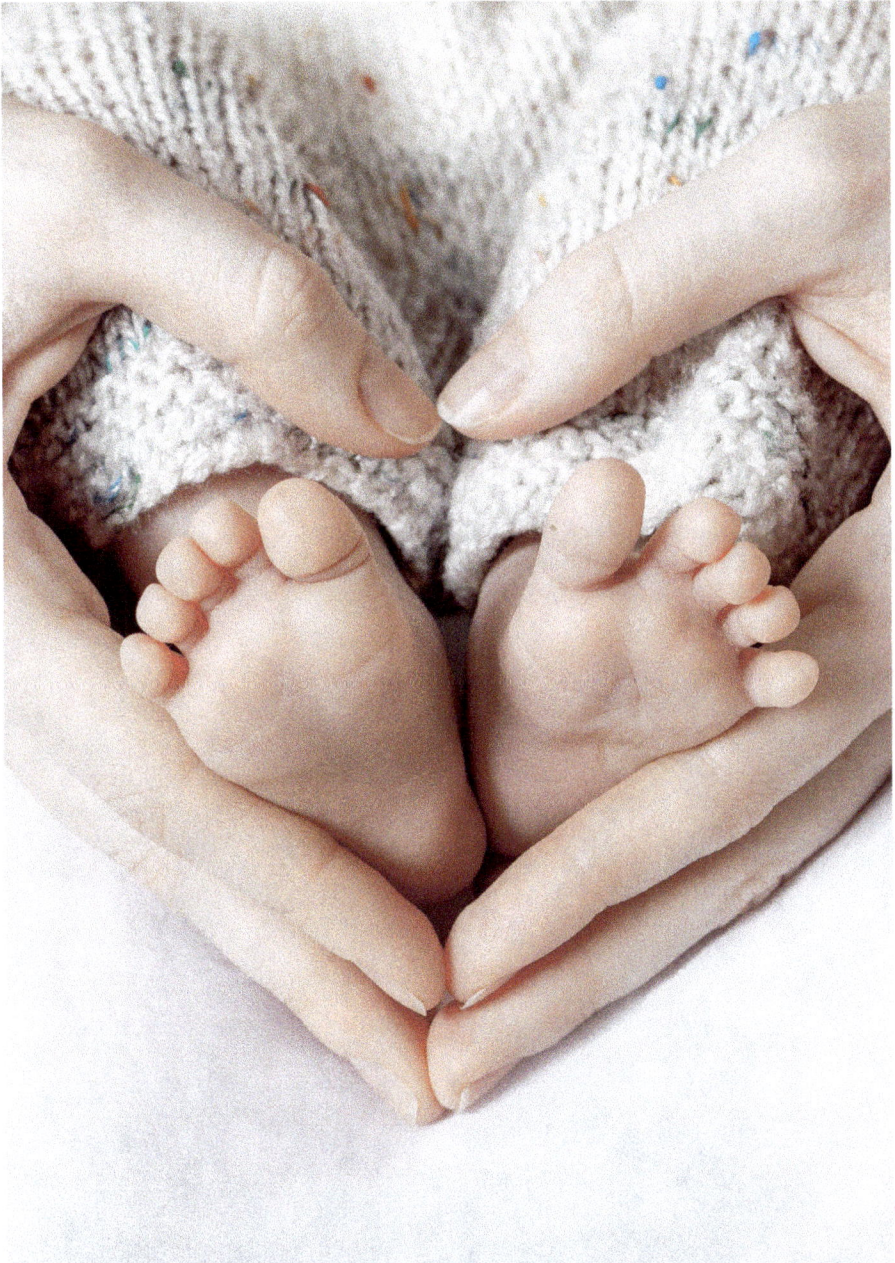

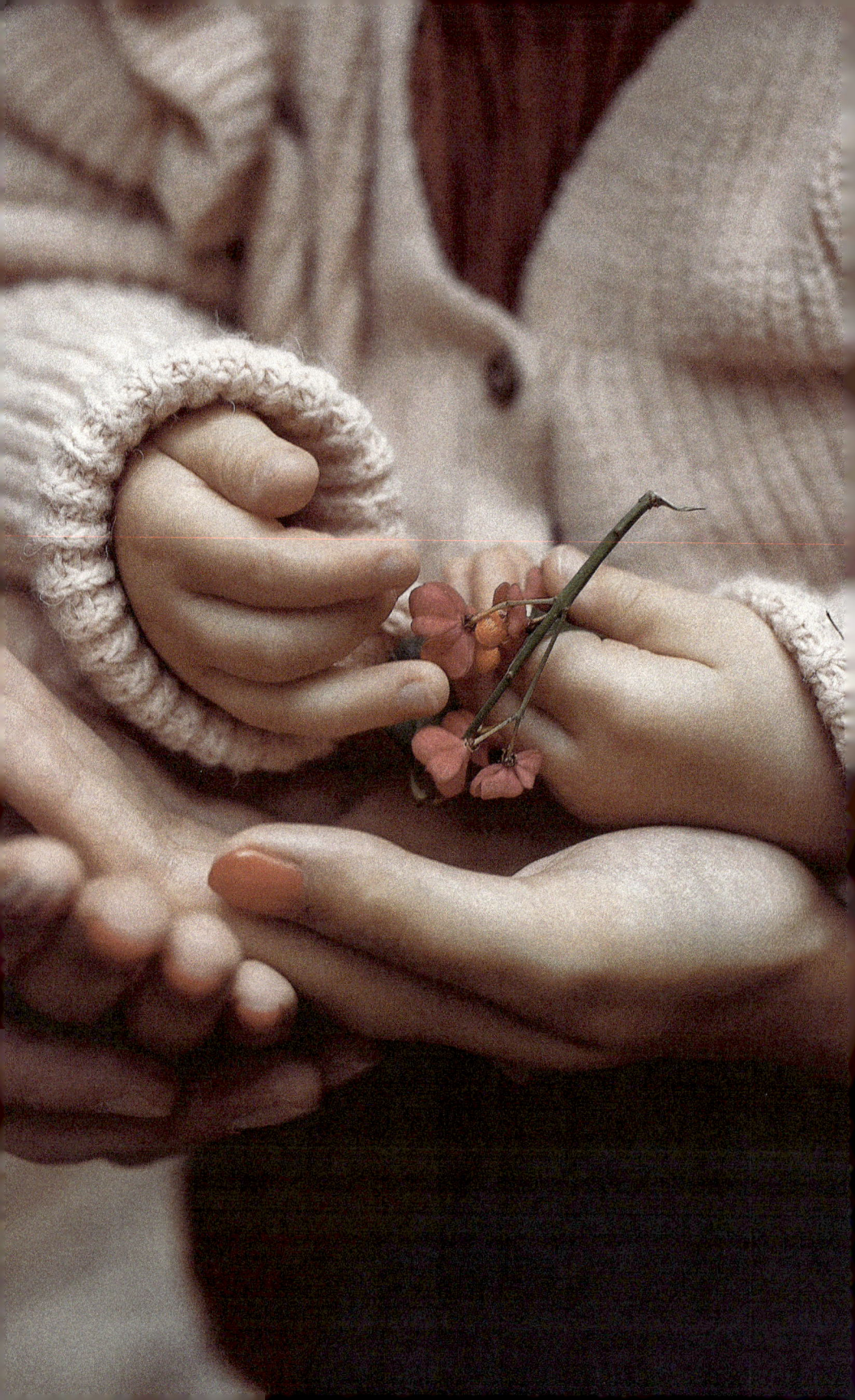

# Chapter 13: A Primer on the Hormones of Childbirth

Your BMP must go through a lot of changes. Her hard-won figure will soon be transformed. Her mobility will decrease. She may experience constant nausea. She's suffering all of this in the name of having a baby with you. So, your best possible move is to attempt to make her pregnancy easier by any means possible.

Find out things she must deal with in her everyday life that you can take off her hands, even if it means a little extra effort on your part. Be considerate of things she can no longer do all the time. If she's having trouble with morning sickness, keep crackers and ginger ale in all parts of the house. Finally, let her know you love her. Plan a good old-fashioned date night, complete with flowers and some well-thought-out plans. It might be a fun time to relive some of those old memories.

### Handling the Hormones

I hate to stereotype, but it requires so much less thought. So, if the following description doesn't jibe with your experience, I apologize in advance. The implantation of the egg into the uterus causes the production of hCG (or beta hCG), the pregnancy hormone. It causes the production of estrogen and progesterone. These hormones are quite necessary for the development of the baby, but like steroids and unprotected sex, they have side effects. As production of the hormones continues, the levels in her body begin to increase. During weeks 5, 6, and 7, pregnancy hormones start making your BMP crazy. Like DEFCON 1 crazy. Typical symptoms include nausea, fatigue, and tender nipples, plus urinating more than your grandfather.

### You Against the Hormones

You as opposed to the hormones are like Spinks against Tyson, Joe against the volcano, and Tiger against monogamy. You have no chance. The pregnancy hormones are just too high. They make her emotions change, and they make her body change. Lots of regular foods she used to enjoy might make her react as if you just cut loose some mighty Taco Bell-driven wind. Her moods may become as unpredictable as a roulette wheel, and you'll have similar odds at predicting them. Fatigue becomes a major issue and her bedtime and dinnertime may start to coincide with one another. But on a positive note, her all-day sickness (we're starting a campaign to rename "morning sickness") may show some signs of slowing down, although for many women it rages on into the second trimester before subsiding. Constipation and flatulence, gifts from your unborn angel, may become significant at these times. Just pretend you're back in freshman year of college with a roommate who has rapidly gained weight, farts all the time, and sleeps a lot. But there is one significant difference. The additional bra size she has earned has you believing this pregnancy may have some advantages after all.

### Chores, Daddy Style

In the beginning, you were just so glad to be pregnant. As your little science project grew, your BMP began to wear down, up to the point where if she was eating at all, she was elbowing seniors out of the way at their favorite Early Bird Special spot so she could get to bed by 6 pm.

Men, in general, show support and affection by providing financially for their families. These people may attempt to help by bringing in cleaning services to knock out those things called chores. But women don't always take kindly to having strangers invade their home. Besides, many times you have these invasive (and expensive) visitors come in to clean only to find they have done everything wrong in the eyes of your significant other. The best, but most unattractive, the solution may be to show support with your actions, even if this includes scrubbing toilets and doing the laundry.

Of all the changes Junior will bring to your schedule, social life, financial life, and sex life, it's the physical changes to your BMP that are starting to be most evident now. Quite a few changes are going on, both inside and out. Let's take a moment to consider some of them.

Yes, Sparky, I know breast enlargement is one of them.

1. Belly. Somewhere around week 12, the baby begins to pooch out. Between months 2 and 3, her uterus will have grown to her belly button. By the end of the whole shooting match, that little miracle will have stretched things out up toward her rib cage.

2. Breasts. I will attempt to keep this part purely as it pertains to the gestation of your future child. Her breasts are preparing to produce milk for the baby. Estrogen, among other hormones, is working to increase the glands that produce this nutritious liquid. During pregnancy, these changes can often lead to breast enlargement (see, I'm biting my tongue). Her breasts may feel slightly firm and are often tender to try to hold back. Your partner may need a bigger bra as this growth progresses. Oh, for God's sake, let the puppies breathe!

3. Heart. Okay, I'm back. Sorry for that unnecessary outburst. Because of the future child taking up residence in Hotel Uterus, your BMP's blood supply will increase by one-third to one-half by the end of her pregnancy. In turn, her heart must work harder to move this blood around. Her heartbeat can change from a usual resting rate of about 70 beats per minute to a comfortable pace of between 80 to 90 beats per minute. Keep this in mind when you're out for your daily twenty-miler with your BMP. She may not be able to keep up with her usual pace.

4. Gastrointestinal system. Those good old hormones are at it again. Some of the same hormones vital to maintaining a healthy pregnancy can also cause nausea and vomiting, along with other GI problems. If the breast enlargement portion got you all hot and bothered, here's the antidote: belching, constipation, and increased flatulence are common during pregnancy. How's that for a cold shower?

5. Skin. The ever-present hormones can cause her skin to show brown patches as additional melanin is produced. There is even individual rashes only pregnant women experience.

So, love her body, whatever the shape or size. Encourage her. Touch her with familiarity, whether it's with a gentle neck rub or holding her hand at the mall. The bottom line is that you want to communicate to her your feelings for her haven't changed or wavered no matter what her shape is in now. All you can hope for is that she'll return the favor as you slowly lose your figure, hair, and all sense of style.

### Managing Weight Gain

Your BMP is going to gain weight. Another human is trapped in there, after all. So, there's some truth to the saying that she's eating for two. But you, on the other hand, are not, so don't act like it. Whether you're eating for one or two, all bodies prefer a healthy diet to a steady stream of chicken wings.

You may be picturing her being all healthy while you continue to plow through a plate of cheese fries. I don't recommend it. It would feel like watching your friends accidentally stumble into a free all-you-can-drink event sponsored by the Swedish Bikini All-Stars on the night you're the designated driver. So, be considerate and behave around her. Moderation in your drinking, especially if it was something she enjoyed before pregnancy, is the prudent course. If the impregnation magic happened after a night of partying, don't pull out the "it reminds me of our night together and our child's conception" speech. She isn't buying it, no matter how great your sales skills. Playing the game this way may even earn you a couple of guilt-free nights out with your BMP's blessing. The keyword is might.

As for smokes, give them up. It's for your good — and your baby's. Secondhand smoke will have your child sounding like a truck driver and rebuilding carburetors before his or her third birthday, not to mention all the other health conditions it can cause or worsen.

As your BMP gains weight with the growth of your seed, you may also gain weight. Don't give us the research about "sympathy weight." Do something good for yourself and eat healthfully with her.

### Pickles and Ice Cream

If you watch enough movies, you'll see a poor father-to-be sent out in the middle of the night because his pregnant wife craves something. You've seen it before, right? The clock shows 2 am., and she shakes the poor boy awake. Invariably, she tells him that he needs to run to the store right now for some bizarre combination of foods. The guy, of course, simply cannot say no to her because she's pregnant. Much humor ensues.

It's true. Many reports that their BMPs craved food from a particular restaurant. Some claim their partners wanted salty foods, while others say it was an ice cream sundae that was in such demand. The medical field hasn't conclusively documented the reasons for these stereotypical cravings. Their theories remain just that. As any man who has been through the process will tell you, it's probably best just to get her what she wants, when she wants it, if humanly possible.

Despite the hype, I've never been asked to run to the store at midnight for pickles and ice cream. Except for that one time in college but nobody was pregnant.

### *Pregnancy Massage*

It's time for the two of you to reconnect. I understand that your secret weapon is the art of seductive massage. I further understand that taking this weapon of mass seduction away from you is like sending a gladiator into the ring without his sword. But alas, I need to de-sword you. Don't try to play amateur masseur here. An incorrect message can trigger contractions. Aromatherapy can also cause problems. Find a massage therapist who is specially trained in massaging pregnant women and give your BMP a gift certificate.

Or better still, take the time to learn what messages you can safely give (ask her doctor). With all the remodeling going on, she's likely to be sore. By likely, I mean 100 percent of pregnant women report feeling this way. Besides, what better way for you two to relax together?

# Chapter 14: Deciding Who Gets to Be in Your Delivery Room

I talk a lot about the mind-body connection because it's important to realize just how much your thoughts and spoken words affect your physical wellbeing. We've already touched on choosing your language carefully, to both reflect what you want to manifest, as well as visualize the ideal birth experience in your mind's eye.

Additionally, you and your birth partner(s) should seek out other parents who are planning or have already had natural births. The easiest way to do this is to seek out local natural birthing resources through your midwife or doula, or by searching online for natural birthing classes in your community. By surrounding yourself with like-minded individuals, you'll increase the support system for you and your partner. Many of us did not grow up in a world where you go against mainstream medical advice, so it is helpful to cultivate a team of positive people who share your views.

It is also important to watch natural birth videos and read natural birth stories. These will help counteract the negative or dramatized visions of labor seen in popular culture. Consider encouraging your partner to watch and/or read with you. (After all, if you as a woman don't have a lot of experience seeing and hearing natural birthing stories, then your partner, especially if he's male, certainly doesn't.)

Similarly, I highly encourage you to watch the movie "The Business of Being Born" if you haven't already. Every woman I interviewed—literally, every one of them—watched this documentary. And I know many partners who were convinced of the benefits of natural birth (and therefore more committed to supporting the woman through one) because of seeing this film. Other powerful documentaries regarding birth, breastfeeding, and early life include "Why Not Home," "The Mama Sherpas," "Birth Story: Ina May Gaskin and The Farm Midwives," "The Beginning of Life," and "The Milky Way."

The tip before, "Choose Your Narrative," and this tip, "Surround Yourself with Positive Support," both encourage you to build up the productive, constructive, optimistic energy around you. One 2009 study even concluded that pregnant women (especially near the end of pregnancy) are better at encoding other people's emotions, particularly those associated with anxiety. Especially with this heightened ability to internalize the stressors of others, it is important to keep a positive company. This is the time to invest only in relationships that help support you and your commitment to natural birth. Avoid those who will compound your fears, tell scary birth stories, or place their own fears and insecurities onto your birth experience.

If this starts to happen, you can politely steer the conversation to a neutral topic like your excitement to meet the baby or becoming a parent. Don't be afraid to cut them off by saying, "I know birth can be challenging, but I'm trying to stay positive, so I don't get wrapped up in fear." Consider easing away from relationships that do not feel supported during this important time. The idea of cutting people out might sound harsh, but you can detach with love by gently letting them know that you don't want to carry any additional worries or stressors. You are already carrying a baby!

Partners sometimes encounter this scare-talk as well. "Man, our house looked like a crime-scene after the homebirth" or "You lose all your freedom when the baby comes." This is because, well, misery loves company. But your partner should also avoid being around such negative talk. What we hear on the outside often becomes our inner dialogue, subliminally. Choose your inputs wisely so you frame your world in rose—but still realistically—colored glasses.

You and your partner want to build a support network and remove yourself from negative influences and generally stressful imagery. I'm talking about you, Game of Thrones. So, respect yourself and your choices enough to walk away from people and things that do not serve you well during this vulnerable and important time.

«For my husband, going to the natural birthing class with me was big for getting us on the same page. Initially he'd said, "That's ridiculous! Why would you want to do the birth without drugs?" But after the class, with all the great information and other committed, intelligent couples, it became a non-issue.»~ Katy, Pennsylvania. Two natural birthing center births.

«One thing that really helps, in terms of being prepared, is to not let people tell you terrible stories. People feel like they need to prepare you by telling you horror stories about their own or other people's experiences, and it's not helpful. It scares people. It makes them anticipate this rough experience regardless of what they're hoping for. So especially for women who are planning a natural birth, which takes extra gumption, you must be more careful of which stories you listen to and seek out the positive ones.»~ Colleen, South Korea, and Italy. Two natural birthing center births.

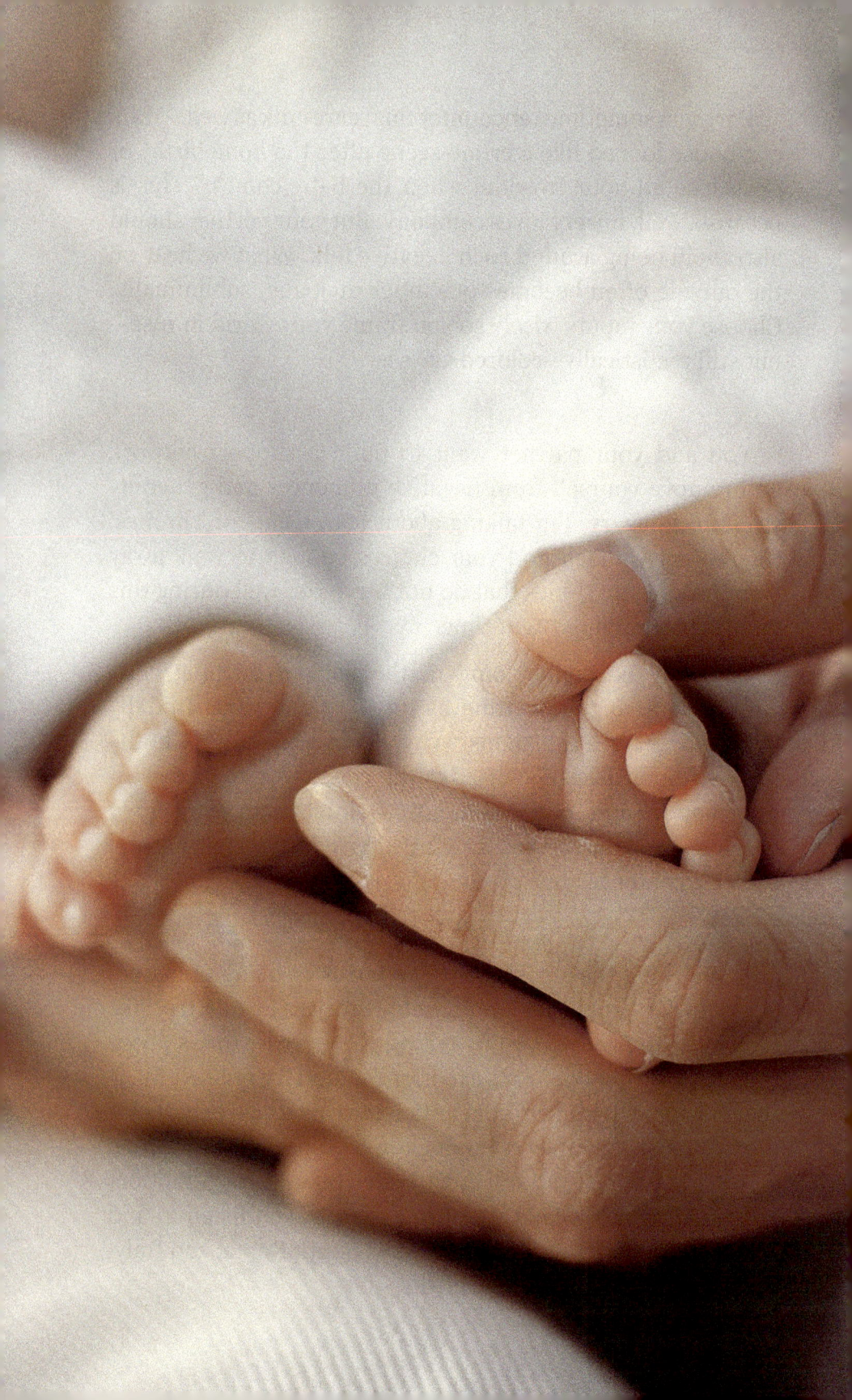

# Chapter 15: The Psychology of Beginning Breastfeeding

### *Milk Ducts, Activate!*

Around day three to five, your milk will change from colostrum to transitional milk. This is a hormonal process triggered by the delivery of your placenta during birth. Some moms will become engorged (super full) at this stage. We are talking breasts so big, so rock hard, so veiny, that they might feel foreign. It's wild, it's a little scary, and yes, it can hurt. These boobs have a job to do now, though, and they are taking it very seriously. (This may also be about the time you tell your partner to never, ever touch them again. That's a normal reaction.)

Often, engorgement happens in the middle of the night. You may wake up to find yourself in a puddle of milk. That's supernormal. (By the way, it's also normal if you don't get engorged. Some moms experience a more gradual transition.) If you find yourself uncomfortably engorged, do not use pumping or heat as your primary means of relieving engorgement. This will compound the issue, making your breasts fuller and more uncomfortable over time. Instead, apply cold compresses (bags of frozen peas or corn work great) to your breasts for 15 minutes a couple of times an hour, and continue to feed baby on demand. Avoid applying cold right before the feed. If you are so full that no milk will come out, then apply warm compresses right before the breastfeed for a few minutes. The initial engorgement should resolve in 24 to 48 hours. If it lasts longer, reaches out to a lactation consultant.

## Standard Equipment:

- **BREASTS**: Mammary glands extending from the front of the chest, which produce milk in pubescent and adult females.

- **LOBULES**: Glands where breast milk is produced.

- **DUCTS**: Network of tubes that carry the breast milk from the lobules to the nipple.

- **AREOLA**: Circle of darker skin around the nipple. It typically gets darker during pregnancy, which may be a visual clue to help the baby find the breast.

- **MONTGOMERY GLANDS**: Small glands around the areola (they look like little pimples!) that secrete a natural oil, which cleans and lubricates the nipple and areola. The oil also contains antibacterial properties to protect the breasts from infection, and it smells like amniotic fluid to help the baby find the breast. (Mother Nature is really giving baby lots of clues to find that breast!)

### *Breast Activation Day*

Your body has never accomplished as much in one day as the day you gave birth. No matter how your baby exited your body or where you were when that happened, the biological machine that is you just succeeded in performing the impressive task of birthing a human (or humans). And it's not done yet. It's time to ACTIVATE!

The moments immediately following birth are crucial to setting your next programmed task—lactation—into motion.

Whether you give birth vaginally or via C-section,

ideally your baby will be placed skin-to-skin on your chest immediately, if baby and mom are both healthy and stable.

The first hour of a baby's life is also known as the "golden hour" and can be a very important time. It's ideal that mom and baby are not separated unless medically necessary. All measurements and observations can be done while you are holding your baby. If the baby needs to be taken from you for anything, including a bath, request that it be put off for at least an hour.

Please know that if you missed out on the golden hour and immediate skin-to-skin contact, you are not destined to fail at breastfeeding—just feed as soon as you and baby are together again.

### *Bonding Post-Birth*

Bonding with a baby is not one moment in time, but rather it's a continuous experience. If you didn't have the birth you planned for, or if you were separated from your baby, it doesn't mean that you won't have a meaningful bonding experience.

Skin-to-skin—laying baby on your chest so they can smell you, hear your heartbeat, and feel your warmth—is a very powerful way of bonding. If the baby is already clean and bundled in blankets and an onesie, you can undress them and remove your top so that you can place them on your chest. Cover baby with a blanket if necessary.

At home, babywearing can be a great way to get in lots of skin-to-skin, keeping your baby happy and your arms free!

Some moms enjoy a "re-birthing bath" once they're both cleared to take a bath. This tends to be especially powerful for moms who didn't birth their baby or who didn't have the birth they planned for.

Recipe for a "re-birthing bath":

- Draw a shallow, lukewarm bath.

- Mom gets in the bath first.

- Either mom or a support person puts the baby in the water on their back (being careful to keep baby's ears out of the water).

- Mom or support person holds the baby and allows the baby to "float" in the water (this is meant to re-create the womb experience).

- Mom can talk to, sing to, or gently stroke baby.

- When the baby is relaxed, place baby tummy down on mom's tummy in the water. The baby may crawl toward the breast and may latch and start breastfeeding.

### Baby in the NICU

Your baby going to the NICU (neonatal intensive care unit) can be a very stressful situation. It may be something you planned for, or it may be a surprise.

Know that there is a team in the hospital ready to support you, including doctors, nurses, lactation consultants, social workers, and caseworkers. There's usually a pumping room in the NICU where you can pump while you're there with your baby. There are also lactation consultants who are available to meet with you, answer your questions, and assist you with breastfeeding.

You may find it helpful to connect with other NICU moms, either in person or over social media. If you have a partner or local family and friends, consider taking shifts at the hospital so you have time to take care of yourself.

### NICU tips:

• If possible, start pumping within six hours of baby's birth.

• In the first few days, hand expression can be more efficient at removing colostrum than an electric pump.

• Pump both breasts every 3 hours for 15 minutes to establish and protect your milk supply.

• Use a hospital-grade pump.

• Ask staff for breast milk storage guidelines and protocols for their facility.

• Try to do lots of skin-to-skin with the baby whenever possible.

• Understand it may take time for the baby to learn to feed at the breast.

• Request that a lactation consultant comes see you in the NICU when you are ready to start breastfeeding.

• Connect with other NICU parents for community, resources, and information, both in person and online.

### *The First Breastfeed*

Given time, your baby could find your breast all on their own by army-crawling their way there from your chest. That's their instinct. Even if you place them on the breast yourself shortly after giving birth, you'll both benefits.

The skin-to-skin contact and suckling will trigger hormones that help your uterus contract, and there is research that finds breastfeeding within the first hour of life can lead to longer breastfeeding relationships.

Your breasts will not feel any fuller or different than they did while you were pregnant at this point. Prior to giving birth, you may notice a clear or golden liquid coming from your breasts. (Don't worry if you don't notice it, though.) This is colostrum, and it's exactly what your newborn needs right now.

A full serving of colostrum is just dropping—about 2 to 10 milliliters. Your baby's stomach is very small and only needs that little bit to fill up. Look at the stomach size comparison chart here.

Newborns should nurse for a minimum of 8 to 12 times every 24 hours. From there, you'll want to time feedings from the beginning of one to the beginning of the next, aiming to breastfeed every 2 to 3 hours.

It's very important that you put the baby to your breast as often as you can. The hormones your body produces every time your baby latches are what signal further milk production.

### *How to Break A Latch?*

Once baby has a solid latch, getting them off your nipple isn't as simple as pulling them away. In fact, that's not advisable at all.

Instead, you need to insert your finger between their gums, break the seal, and scoop your nipple out of their mouth. This is one of many reasons why it's a good idea to wash your hands before you breastfeed. You might also want to keep your nails short and polish-free.

If your baby bites down on your nipple while nursing, quickly break the latch and, with a firm tone, let baby know that hurt. Take a break from nursing. Don't smile or make it a game, or the biting might continue. For more on biting and teething, see here.

## Tracking Feeds

For the first few weeks, keep a daily (24-hour) log of:

- The number of breastfeeds
- How long the breastfeeds are
- Which side(s) you used
- How many bottles
- How many ounces in the bottle?
- How many wet diapers
- How many stools

There are apps available for your phone that make tracking easier and allow tracking to be shared between multiple people.

Of course, the old-school way of writing stuff down in a notebook also works. If you go low-tech, one way to keep track of which breast is up next on the menu is to wear a bracelet or even a hair tie on your wrist on whatever side you last nursed. Once you latch baby to the opposite side at the next feeding, switch the bracelet over to that wrist.

When you meet with your pediatrician or the lactation consultant, they will ask for these numbers. When you are sleep-deprived, each day starts to blur with the next one, so documenting feedings and diaper changes as they happen will make your life easier.

Many moms wonder if they should use one breast or two during each feed. The hospital will recommend you feed the baby for 10 minutes on each side every time you feed. Once your milk transitions, most moms do a full feed on one side and offer the second side as "dessert." Sometimes, the baby may want only one side, and sometimes the baby may want both. Alternate the breast you start with to ensure that both breasts receive equal stimulation.

# Part 6: The Fourth Trimester: Recovery, Adaptation, and Ambivalence in Your First Trimester of Motherhood

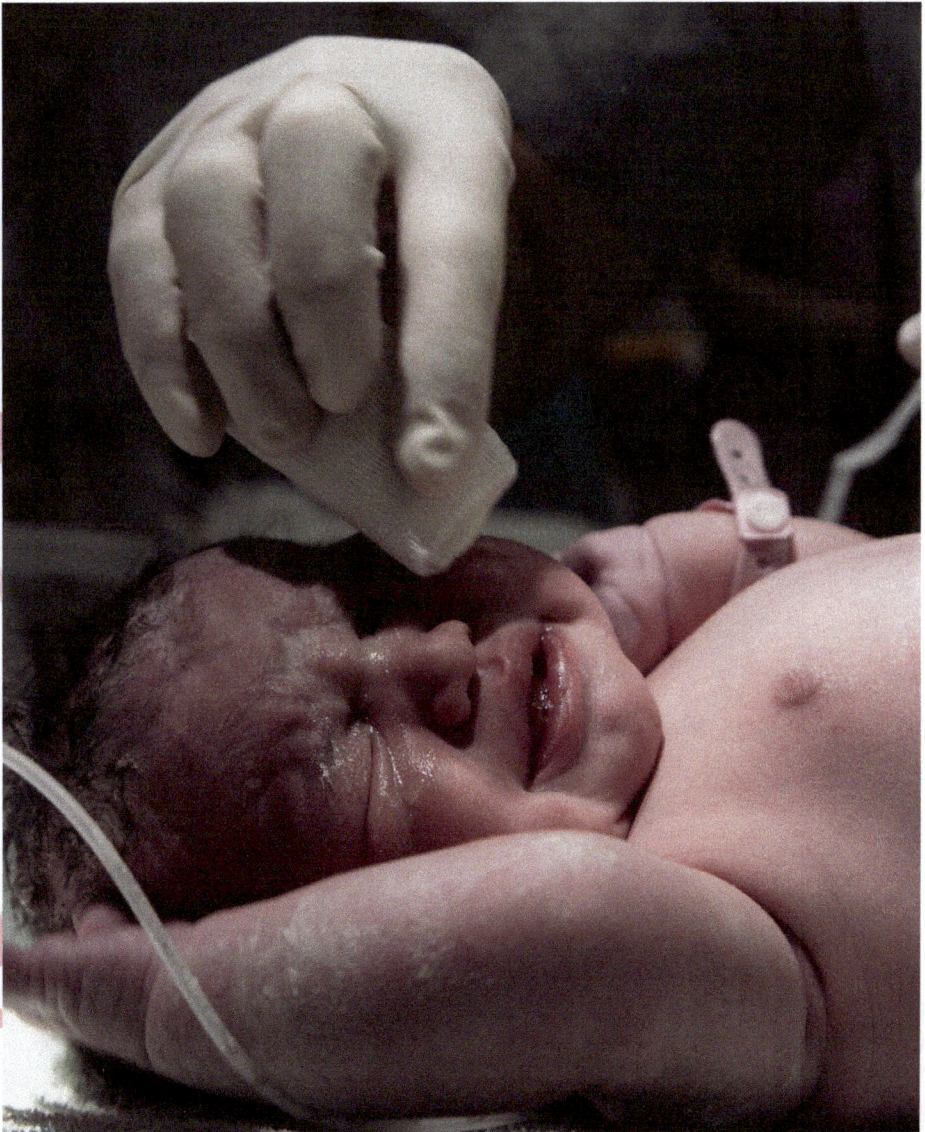

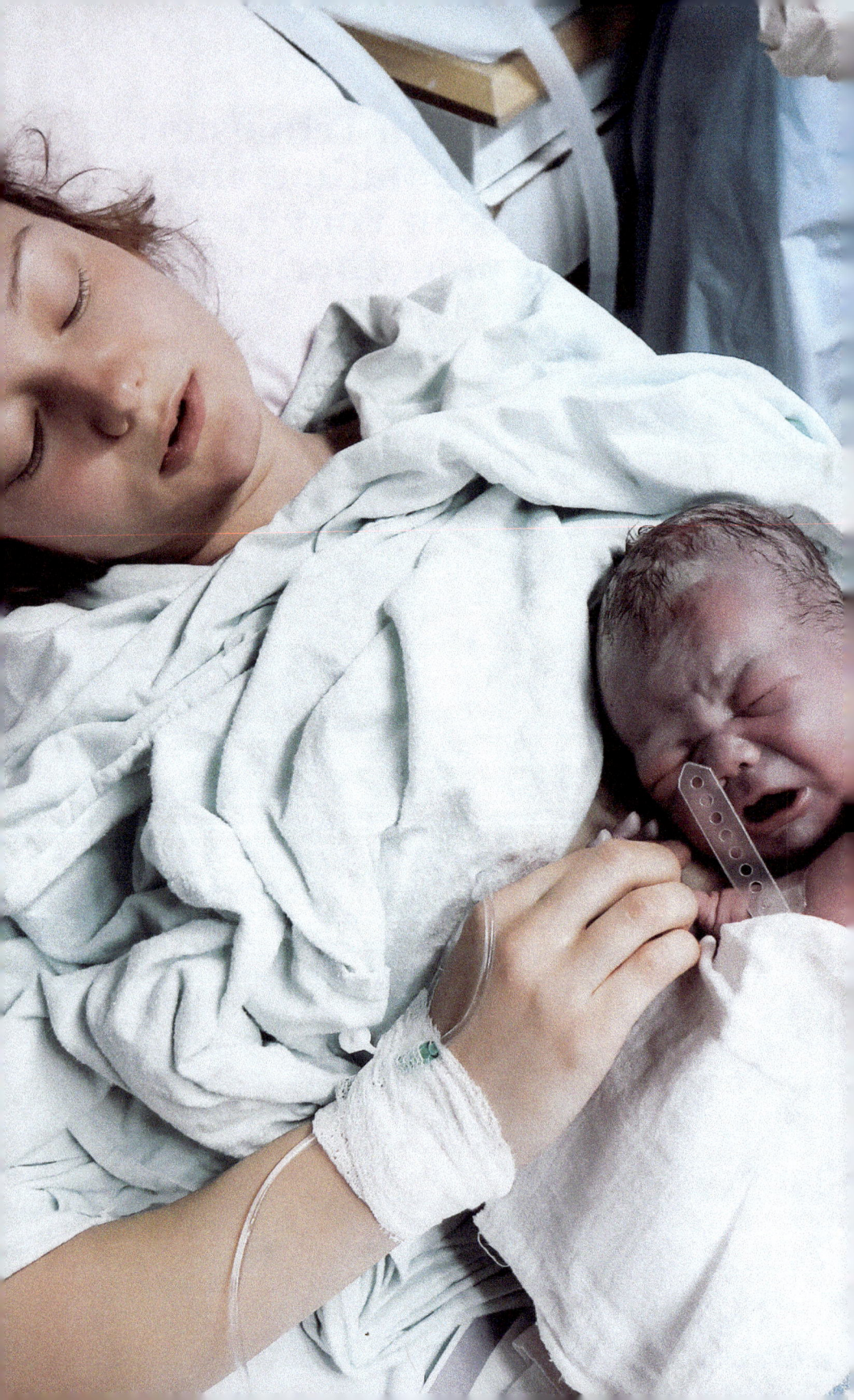

# Chapter 16: The Intense Experience of Being Alone with Your Baby

O nce you bring your baby home from the hospital, your daily way of life is going to change. While you might return to work at your same job and spend time together as a couple, you now have a wonderful new addition to include in your life. Living with a child changes a lot about the typical routine shared by two adults. There are plenty of new tasks for you to learn to make your baby feel comfortable and safe.

Most of these things are probably what you have already thought about, but now you are going to learn how to execute them effectively. Like anything that relates to mothering, you are going to become better at it as you practice it. By tuning into your maternal instincts, you will be able to create a beautiful life for your child.

## *Bathing and Personal Hygiene*

When bathing a newborn, remember that this is something that only needs to happen once or twice a week, and only if the umbilical cord has fallen off. If your baby still has their cord, you will have to give them sponge baths. This is because frequent bathing can dry out their fragile skin. As your baby gets older, you can increase this frequency. Bathing your baby can be a very nerve-wracking experience, but you are going to be great at it. No matter what, you should never walk away from your baby while they are bathing. They need constant supervision, even while they are in their infant tub. To get started, make sure that you have an infant bathtub (it will go in the sink or in your regular bathtub), mild soap that does not contain irritants, a soft washcloth, two bath towels, a change of diaper and clothing, and a baby hairbrush.

Once your little one is in the tub, you can follow these simple steps:

- Wash their face with plain water;

- Clean their eyes by wiping away any debris in the corners;

- Clean the surfaces of their nose and ears (avoiding internal contact with water);

- Wash their body with mild soap;

- Rinse them with plain water;

- Pat your baby dries with a clean towel;

- Take the baby into your arms and massage the shampoo into their head;

- Rinse their head thoroughly to avoid any scalp build-up;

- Towel dry their hair and then brush it with a soft baby brush;

- Dress your baby in a diaper and appropriate clothing;

### Nail Care

Keep your baby's fingernails trimmer to prevent them from scratching themselves. If there are any rough edges, use a baby nail file to smooth them out. To trip your baby's fingernails safely, hold the skin away from the nail and cut straight across with a pair of baby nail clippers. If you know you need to trim their nails, do so after a bath because the nails will be softer and easier to trim. Another suggestion is to trim their nails while they are sleeping. Your baby might get fussy if they are away while you try to trim them.

Your baby's nails will grow fast, but you do not have to trim them too often. You should make sure that the nails are long enough to cut safely without accidentally cutting any of their surrounding skin. If you need to supplement, you can put mittens over your baby's hands to prevent them from scratching themselves. This is especially helpful while they sleep, as they will not have any control over how they might move their hands.

### *Ear Care*

There is not too much that you will have to do for your baby's ears. In the bath, you are already going to be cleaning the surfaces of their ears, and this is a perfectly adequate way to clean them. You do not want to stick any cotton swabs or other cleaning devices inside of their ear canals because this could rupture your baby's eardrums. Their ears are very fragile, and they can easily be injured. The same can be said about cotton balls—don't use them on your baby's ears, even the surfaces. Residue from these cotton balls can become lodged inside your baby's ears.

If you notice that your baby is constantly trying to touch their ears and crying, this could be an indication that they have an ear infection. Babies commonly develop ear infections, so this is no need for too much concern. As soon as you notice your baby displaying this behavior, you can take them to the doctor and an antibiotic will be prescribed. Babies tend to be very susceptible to ear infections, and many develop multiple during their time as an infant.

### Nose Care

Your baby's nose is likely to get messy, but it should not be hard to clean if you handle it right away. For any mucus, clean it gently with a tissue. For anything that is dried up, you should soak a washcloth in warm water to be able to clean it without hurting your baby. They are likely going to squirm when you try to clean their nose but know that it should not cause them pain if you work gently.

In some cases, using a nasal syringe is necessary. Your baby does not know how to blow their nose, so they can become congested very easily. The nasal syringe consists of a small bulb that works with air pressure to remove any build-up inside of your baby's nose. The nurses at the hospital used this device when your baby was first born. You shouldn't always have to use the nasal syringe, but it is helpful to keep one around just in case.

### Diaper Changes and Dressing Baby

Changing your baby's diapers is something that you are going to be able to master efficiently. At first, the concept might be foreign to you, causing you to move slower. Be patient with yourself. You will get better at this the more that you do it. When you suspect that your baby needs a diaper change, their behavior will usually confirm this. They might cry or appear visibly uncomfortable. If they have peed in their diaper, it is going to look much denser and have a thicker feel to it from the outside. If your baby has pooped, you are likely going to smell it. You can gently pull back the waistband of the diaper to confirm if your baby has used the bathroom.

Your hygiene matters a great deal when you are changing your baby's diaper. You need to make sure that your hands are washed before you get started. This will ensure that no germs are being spread to your baby. After you finish, of course, you will also wash your hands. When it comes to changing your baby's diaper, you just need to rely on your common sense. Do not use any harsh or perfumed products on your baby that will cause irritation. You will want to be as gentle as you can, too.

Before setting your baby down on the changing pad, make sure that you have your new diaper, wipes, trash can, diaper cream, and any soothing powder at hand. Once you place your baby down on the changing pad, you will not have the opportunity to walk away. After opening your baby's diaper, remove the dirty diaper by gently grabbing both your baby's feet and removing the diaper from underneath them. If your baby has pooped, you can use the clean upper half of the diaper to wipe away the first bit of poop. Then, throw the diaper in the trash.

Take a baby wipe and clean your baby from front to back to avoid infection. You might have to use a couple of wipes if your baby pooped. After ensuring that your baby is fully cleaned, apply any necessary diaper rash cream or powders. Put their new diaper on after this. You will do this by lifting your baby by holding onto their feet gently, and then you will slide their clean diaper underneath them. Once everything has been lined up and adjusted, you can fasten the diaper.

Your baby's diaper should be changed approximately every two to three hours. Of course, this depends on the baby. This gives you a good guideline for how often you should be checking on your baby's diaper, either way. If they are not dirty yet, you can check back again in another hour. Each time that you change your baby's diaper gives you the chance to care for their umbilical cord. Not much needs to be done to it, but you can soak a cotton ball in warm water and wipe away any dry or sticky substances from the perimeter of the cord. After cleaning, pat the area dry with a cloth.

When it comes to changing your baby's clothing, you are going to rely on your common sense again. If your baby soils themselves or gets their clothing dirty in any other way, you can change them to keep them comfortable. Most infant clothing unbuttons or unzips all the way down, allowing you the chance to get their limbs into it easily. If you are putting on a shirt that does not unfasten, place your baby's arms in the armholes gently. You should not have to move your baby into an uncomfortable position to do this. Next, take the hole where their head goes and stretch it out slightly, ensuring that there is plenty of room to put the shirt on without covering your baby's face for a prolonged period. This should easily allow you to get their head in the shirt and then straighten up the bottom half of it.

Make sure that your baby's bottoms are not too tight. While the clothing might fit them perfectly, know that a diaper is bulky, and it will take up more room. If your baby is experiencing discomfort or fussiness when they wear certain clothing, this might be an indication that you need to size up to give them more room for their crotch and legs. Clothing that is too tight can also lead to diaper rash because of the way that it presses into the skin, so always be cautious about this. You can ensure that your baby's clothing is not too tight if it does not leave any marks on your baby's skin. Marks that outline the stitching are an indication that the clothing is digging into your baby.

### *Bonding*

When you have your baby, you are naturally going to expect a wonderful and instantaneous bond with them. This is your child, a part of you that you grew inside of your stomach for nearly a year. It seems obvious that the connection is strong, but this is not always the case. It is normal if your baby does not seem incredibly attached to you at first. Bonding can take time because it is such an individualized process. Do not panic if you feel your baby "doesn't like you." Surely, they do, and they will learn how to show it as they develop more ways to do so. This does not make you a bad mother or a terrible parent if your baby does not immediately take to you. Much like yourself, your baby has just been through a very long and confusing process.

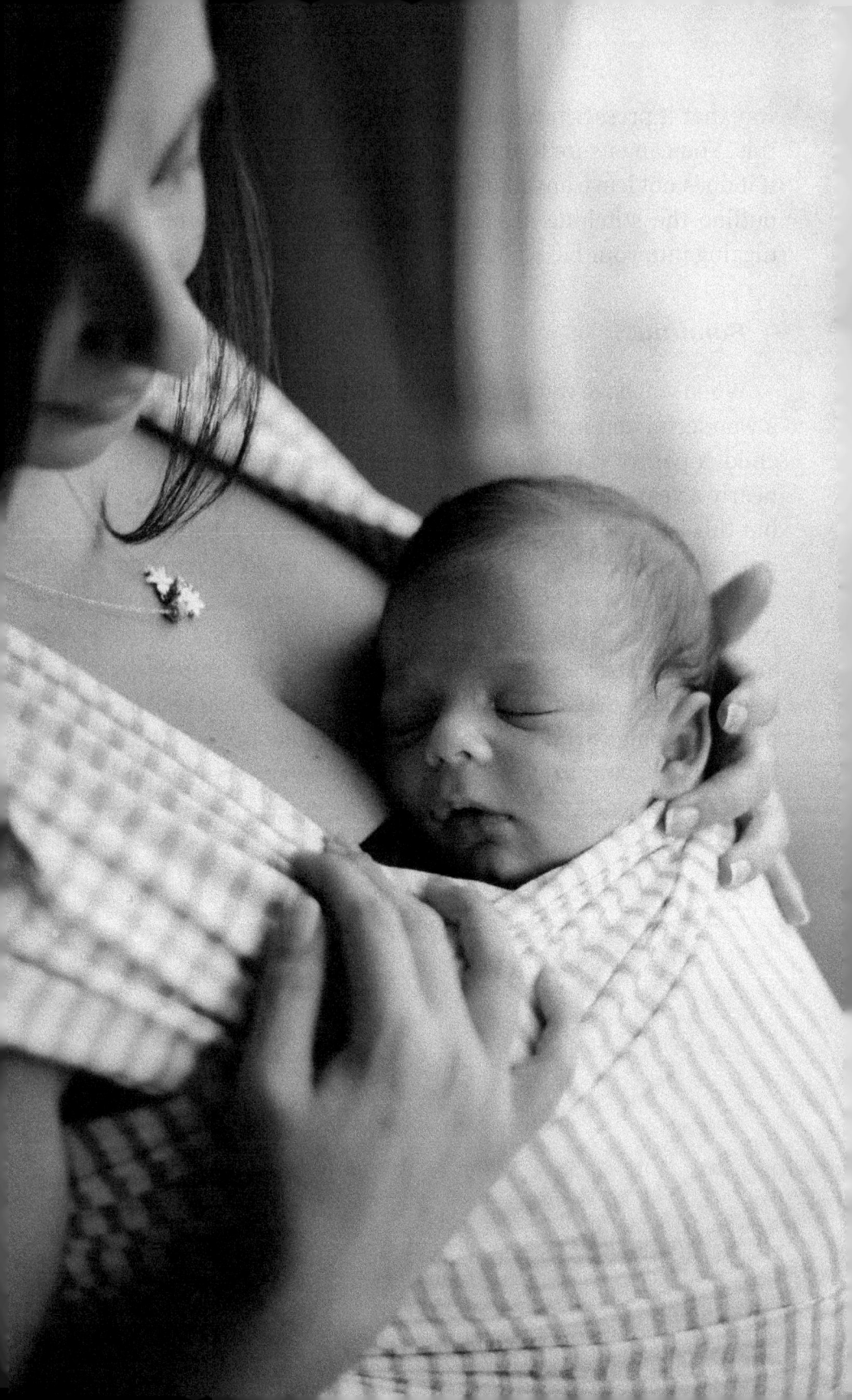

# Chapter 17: How to Preserve (Or Develop) Self-Care for Mothers

When you have a baby, it is the end of the person you once knew and the beginning of you as a mother. In a way, the birth of your child also signals the birth of you as a mother. And in these following months you can choose how to define yourself and reinvent that as many times as you'd like.

The unfortunate reality is, as you enter motherhood, our society asks that you relinquish any idea of autonomy—any idea of being anything more than a mother. However, it's important that you continue to seek out the things that bring joy to your life and that you set time aside to really focus on how you want to define yourself. Yes, you're a mother, but that isn't where the definition of you as a whole person ends.

You must tend to yourself. Your child demands that you are present, which makes the temptation to disconnect from yourself at the end of a long day much more tempting.

When I was in the thick of it in the early weeks postpartum, I'd roll out my yoga mat and take a savasana (corpse pose). As I lay there, I would envision the earth coming up to meet me. Letting my weight sink in, I visualized the great Mother Earth's energy holding me up. At that moment I was grounded, and I felt supported. I recommend this to women in my practice and would encourage you to try sinking into Mother Earth's supportive energy, especially when you feel tempted to disconnect.

### *Engaging Your Creative Center*

Your pelvis is the home of your sacral chakra and your creative energy. When you are tapped into this space you can be more creative with problem-solving the challenges that arise.

### Sacral Chakra Meditation:

Coming into a comfortable seated position, feel the weight of your sit bones on the earth. Visualizing the tailbone as a root, let it drop down and connect into the earth.

Placing your hands over your womb space, close your eyes and begin to send your breath into your pelvis. At first, observe without judgment what comes up as you begin to explore this space.

As you breathe, visualize that earth energy drawing up into the pelvis. Let it swirl and fill your space.

Placing an imaginary filter above your head, draw in a beautiful golden light and let it meet that earth energy in your pelvis. Allow them to swirl, connect, and integrate.

Imagine this energy washing through the pelvis, allowing anything that is not serving you to drop down that root and surrender it to the earth.

This is your space, fill it with what you desire in your life and release anything that you no longer wish to keep.

To close, visualize closing off the light energy and releasing all to the highest good. Take a final deep breath and as you exhale, bow forward. Inhale and on the exhale return to seated.

### Feel like you have no time for this?

At any time, you can simply place a hand on the front of your pelvis and another on your back, just over the sacrum. Send your awareness into this space, even if just briefly. By building this connection you strengthen your ability to drop into a grounded space when life becomes hectic or stressful.

As women, we can store a lot of past grief or traumas that can be released or ignited with birth. Meeting with a pelvic floor therapist or intuitive counselor can help you transition and process the shifts that have evolved after childbirth.

### Are you meeting your basic needs?

Give yourself one point for each of the following:

\_\_\_\_ I eat regular meals and avoid skipping meals and snacks.

\_\_\_\_ I take the time to chew my food well.

\_\_\_\_ I rest often, especially when I feel tired.

\_\_\_\_ I drink fluids throughout the day.

\_\_\_\_ I move my body regularly.

\_\_\_\_ I sleep in a dark room.

\_\_\_\_ I spend time in the sunshine at least three days per week.

\_\_\_\_ I cuddle, hug, or engage in physical touch daily.

\_\_\_\_ I am gentle, loving, and forgiving with myself.

\_\_\_\_ I make time for a shower or bath most days of the week.

\_\_\_\_: Total

If you find yourself with a score of 7 or less, it is time to recruit some help and make a strategy to meet these needs. You are an important and integral part of your family and friends' lives. You must take care of your own health if you are going to be 100% present for those who you care for.

Beyond the basics, you deserve to thrive.

It is not indulgent to care for yourself. Repeat. It is not indulgent to care for yourself, to spend time doing the things you enjoy or to take a break to fill your heart with joy.

Life is more than feedings, naps, burping, diaper changes... you get the idea. It is easy to slip into the role of mom and forget that you are a woman with needs. You will be so much happier if you focus on staying connected with those things that bring you joy. And you'll be a better mom too!

As a working mom, I know all too well how difficult it can be to make time for yourself. I want to share with you a few of my favorite "mini-spa" rituals that I use when I need a little pampering but am short on time.

### When Isn't Sleep Enough?

You've probably heard it multiple times— "sleep when the baby sleeps." This is great advice, but sometimes, sleeping when the baby sleeps isn't enough.

Exhaustion, low mood, anxiety, joint pain, and cold hands and feet are likely signs of larger underlying issues. Hypothyroidism, adrenal fatigue, B12 deficiency anemia, iron deficiency anemia, and autoimmune disease may be contributing to your symptoms.

If you feel like your fatigue goes beyond what should be

expected in motherhood you should speak with your doctor to have a thorough workup. With an exam, complete history and proper laboratory work, your doctor should be able to identify the cause of your exhaustion.

Autoimmunity, a condition in which your immune system mistakenly attacks your own body tissue, can be triggered by childbirth. The symptoms are often difficult to differentiate and may wax and wane for many months and sometimes years. It is important that you seek help from a qualified medical professional who is willing to listen to your story and partner with you to understand what the cause of your symptoms is.

If you suspect something is wrong, don't delay care. Trust your instincts. Addressing autoimmunity early can help you prevent the development of more serious conditions.

### *Natural Remedies to Increase Energy*

Nutritional Supplementation. If you are found to be low in iron, vitamin B12, or other nutrients your fatigue will be amplified. Continuing your prenatal vitamins can help guard against deficiencies, but blood work may be necessary to determine if you have a deficiency or anemia.

Legs Up the Wall (Viparita Karani). This simple yoga pose can be incredibly rejuvenating. Sit close to a wall with the right side of your body touching. As you begin to lay down, allow your legs to move up the wall until they are resting comfortably against it. You can also place a pillow or bolster under your hips to add support.

Rest Often. More than just sleep, whenever possible put your feet up and relax.

Eat Well, Eat Often. Skipping meals or eating processed foods and added, processed sugar will cause your energy to crash and trigger hormone imbalance.

Nurse with Baby Near. Co-sleeping or having a bassinet near your bed can make night feedings less disruptive to your sleep.

Accept Help. Having a baby is a lot of work. If someone offers help, please accept it. There is no shame in not being able to do it all. No one should have to do it all.

Ask for Help. If you need help, you need help. The only way your loved ones will know how to best help you is for you to let them know what you need.

Be Gentle with Yourself. Negative thoughts about your abilities or your life are draining. You're doing an awesome job and even when it doesn't feel that way, please be gentle with yourself.

Be a Team. You and your partner need to communicate and work together. If you don't have someone you are partnering with, I urge you to consider hiring a postpartum doula or connecting with someone else in your life that can help you.

Avoid Dehydration. Staying hydrated has numerous

benefits, including sustained energy.

Choose Healthy Snacks. When you are feeling low, chocolate, potato chips, and easy energy dense foods sound appealing. However, any boost in energy they provide is temporary and you will crash.

Go for a Walk. Yes, I know this seems like a strange recommendation, but even a short gentle walk can help raise your energy and mood.

Fix Nutrient Deficiencies. Vitamin B12, iron, vitamin D, and other nutrients can be tested for and supplemented if necessary.

Ashwagandha Tincture. 2 droppers full twice daily as needed for a pick me up.

I cannot express enough how important it is to address the root cause of your fatigue. If your fatigue is due to a deeper issue, these practices will be helpful, but will not be enough to properly restore your energy and vitality.

### *Nourishing Your Body: Nutrition for New Moms*

Your nutrition is just as important after birth as it was during pregnancy. It may be tempting to jump into a diet as soon as possible with the hopes of losing weight and regaining your pre-baby body. However, I strongly urge you to focus less on weight loss and more on rebuilding your nutrient stores and supplying the most nutrient-dense breast milk to your baby.

I know it's hard to have the extra weight your body gained during pregnancy without the adorable baby bump on the front to go with it. But that weight serves a purpose—it protects you and serves as an energy storehouse for you and baby.

So, while there's nothing wrong with wanting to regain your pre-baby body, we're going to focus instead on optimizing every cell in your body.

Breastfeeding your infant places higher caloric energy and nutrient demands on your body. Your body is providing fuel to a quickly growing human. Your baby is growing faster and is moving more than they were in the womb, which means they need more nutrition from you. The recommended intake for micronutrients is based on what is excreted through your breast milk, although your needs may be higher if you have an underlying condition or are healing from a very traumatic birth.

# Part 7: The First Year of Motherhood

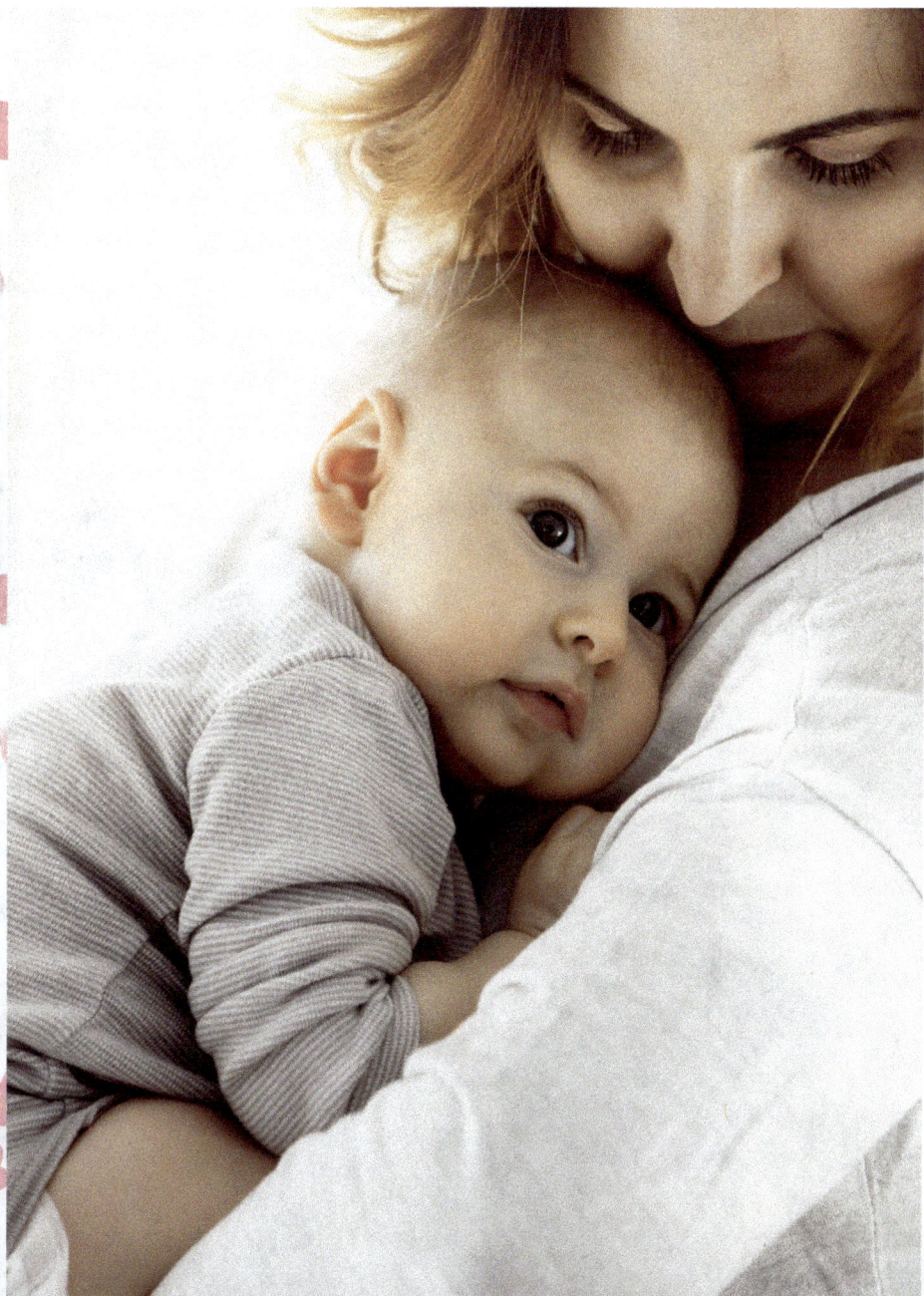

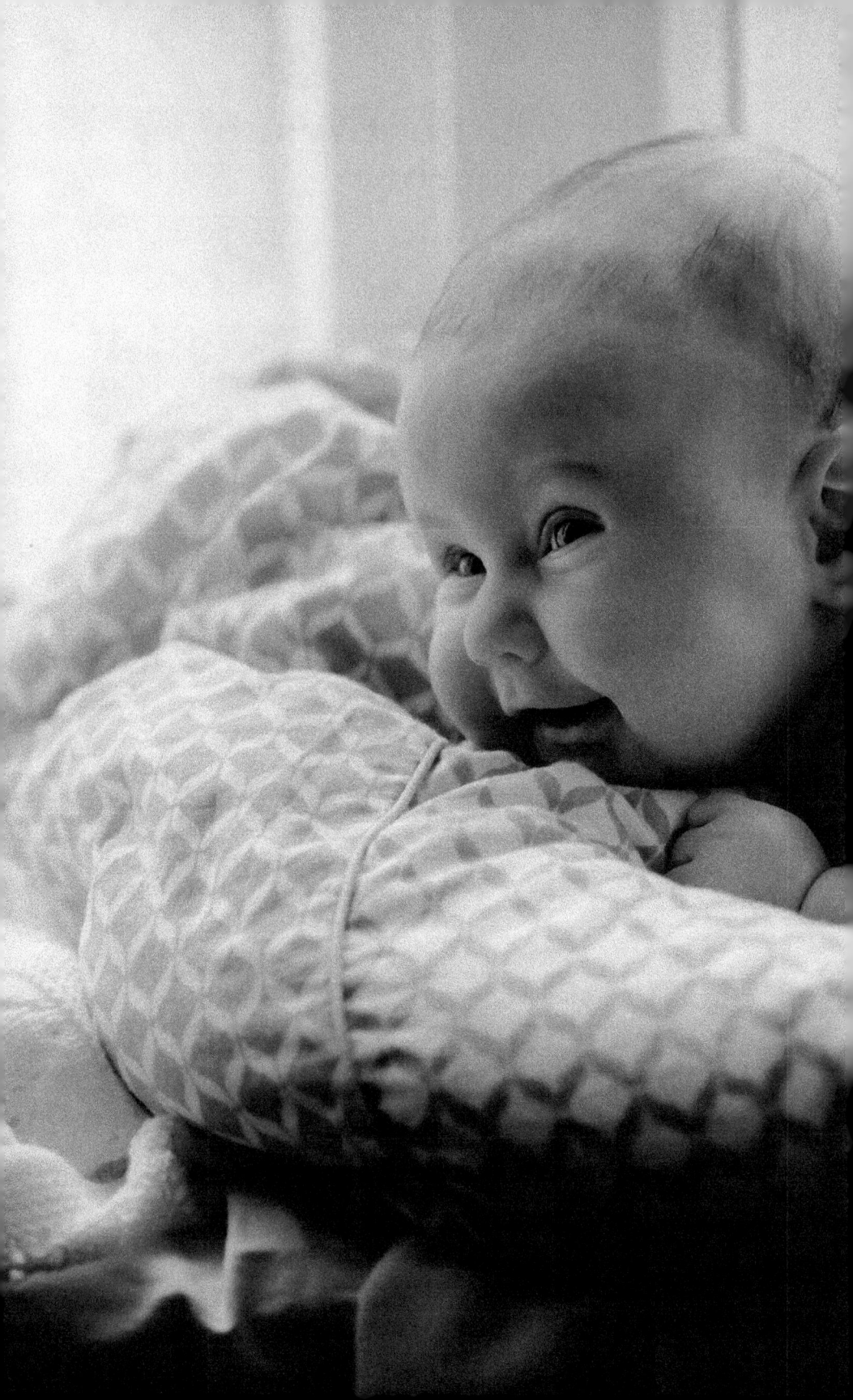

# Chapter 18: Emotionally Wise Approaches to Sleep Training

### *A few notes about sleep training:*

Many parents start to consider sleep-training options around the four-month mark. There are countless infant-sleep professionals and pediatricians who provide advice and guidance for sleep training your baby.

### *You Don't Have to Sleep Train Your Baby*

Whether you get on the sleep-training bus or not, your baby is not going to be a night-waking terror for the rest of your life. It may feel like an eternity, but like all other phases, this will be relatively short-lived.

### These are my friend Matilde's words:

«When my infant was struggling with sleep, I read every word on the Internet about sleep training. All my research taught me one thing: I could parent more effectively, more lovingly, and more joyfully with empathy and comfort. So, I decided to let my baby tell me what felt good. Some nights that meant he nursed himself to sleep, others it meant Dad rocked him for a bit before he drifted off. All of them left us feeling good about the relationship we were building with our little person.

Did my son have a hard time going to sleep without us for a couple of years? Yes.

Did he sleep in my room until he went to kindergarten? Also, yes.

Did I spend hours regretting my choices and beating myself up over the entire thing? Nope. I decided that my own sanity and the general health of our family was what mattered.

But that isn't what worked best for my second son. We did a more traditional sleep-training method with him, and it allowed everyone in the house to get much-needed rest.

Do what is best for your baby and your family. I always tell moms that there are no should in parenting—there are things that work for you and things that don't.»

### *There is No One Way to Sleep Train Your Baby*

If you need to help your baby sleep through the night, there are several methods you may wish to use. Most of us are familiar with some version of Dr. Richard Ferber's famous "cry it out" sleep-training technique. Instead of providing comforts like rocking or feeding baby to sleep, the "cry it out" method encourages parents to put the baby to sleep awake and allow him to cry, offering only brief reassurances by patting and soothing without picking him up. This will allow the baby to learn how to put himself to sleep as opposed to relying on parents to help. Over the years, his original method has received criticism for causing unnecessary stress among parents and infants and, as a result, many have adapted, updated, and reimagined his methods to fit more modern parenting ideas. Dr. Ferber himself made additional modifications to the techniques in his 2006 edition of the book Solve Your Child's Sleep Problems. In it, he encourages parents to adapt his method to fit their own child, parenting style, and circumstances.

While Dr. Ferber's "cry it out" technique seems to be the most well-known sleep-training strategy, there are several methods to help your child achieve restful sleep.

If you're looking for an alternative to "cry it out," the no-cry technique explained by Dr. William Sears may help. In this method, Sears recommends that parents stay engaged with their baby as he transitions to sleep; help the baby find comfort with nursing, rocking, singing, and any other strategies they find comforting. This is a more responsive, intuitive sleep strategy that many believe encourages the parent-child bond and which Sears believes builds trust between the baby and his parents or caregivers.

Regardless of what strategy you employ, remember to keep your eye on the prize: Sleep, for everyone, without all the fuss, is the endgame; how you find your way there is up to you and your baby.

### *Make Sure Everyone is on The Same Page*

Whatever method you decide to go with, it's important that you get all of the baby's caretakers on board. You want baby to understand that going to sleep is not a tumultuous, unpredictable affair. It's a comforting, relieving, safe experience that she should want to have repeatedly.

### *Maintain Flexibility*

This doesn't need to be boot camp. It's totally cooled to allow flexibility in your process and respond to the baby's needs at the moment. Maybe the baby is sick or teething. Maybe she was overstimulated from being handed back and forth between relatives all day. As long as you have a comforting, predictable bedtime routine in place, it's okay to take a break from the sleep-training manual, especially if it's not going well or if your child (or you) could use a change of pace.

# Chapter 19: How Your Relationship to Food Shapes Your Child's Early Feeding

### *Hello to Munching!*

After too many denials at being asked for whatever you are eating, your baby is finally ready to start tasting and even eating! It is truly an important and exciting milestone for mommy and baby, so welcome the new experiences waiting for your baby, but be careful too.

The AAP advises against introducing solids to infants until they're at least six months old and your baby is showing development as predicted, your baby is ready to start solids from around 4-6 months. Starting solids before your baby has even developed the ability to swallow and digest solids isn't safe, and your doctor will also recommend against it.

Indicators that your little one is ready to start solids:

• Your baby should be able to start controlling his head's movement and keep it steady.

• Your baby should also be able to sit unsupported and upright in the feeding chair.

• Your baby will also let you know it is time by reaching for food and opening his or her mouth when a spoon is near their mouth.

### What Do You Start With?

To know how your baby should be starting with the munchies, you should talk to your baby's doctor first. The introduction of solid feedings is usually with unseasoned puree. You'll see most people buying infant cereal, but there's no medical evidence that you must start with packaged cereal, or it provides better provision than normal food mashed for infant digestion.

AAP recommends that you introduce your previously breastfed baby with iron-rich solids like meat such as beef, chicken, or turkey as iron stores start diminishing as they near the 6th month.

You could also alternate meat with pureed sweet potatoes, applesauce, peaches, mashed bananas, or boiled pears.

American Academy of Allergy Asthma and Immunology (AAAI) suggests that giving your baby allergy-inducing foods such as soy, eggs, wheat, fish, or peanut butter around 4-6 months help in preventing food allergies later.

Consult your doctor if your baby has any of the following:

- A sibling with peanut allergies.
- Your baby has eczema.
- Your baby had a previous allergic reaction to a newly introduced food.
- Your baby had a blood test that indicated the possibilities of an allergy.

### *How to Introduce Food to Your Baby?*

Though it is common practice to feed newborns puree or cereal, some parents, however, tend to practice baby-led weaning. The process includes putting soft food in front of your baby and letting your baby choose and feed on his or her own. This process usually leads to spoon-feeding.

For the first few feedings, introduce your baby to puree or cereal in two or three teaspoons right after milk-feeding.

To avoid injuring the gums of your baby, buy the soft-tipped plastic spoons for feeding. If your baby dislikes the sight of the food you're offering and avoids it, be patient. Let your baby smell it and leave it for another day.

If you decide to feed an infant ready-to-eat pouches of baby food, make sure to take out whatever you're feeding the little one into a small plate so you can save the rest for later as there is a high probability of contaminating the food with bacteria from your baby's mouth if you put the same spoon from his or her mouth back into it. Do not keep opened baby food for more than two days.

If you decide to start feeding with cereal, dilute the food and start it off with one teaspoon. If you feel it's too soon to give your baby that too, add just a bit of breast milk or formula milk to it so your baby can warm up to the idea of new food. You can gradually make the cereal more viscous over time once your baby is familiar and comfortable with the food.

Do not add solids to your baby's life immediately. Spread the process over a few days, starting with a teaspoon and gradually increase it till it to two feedings a day. Your baby will need time to understand the concept of swallowing, so be careful, keep your baby upright, and be patient.

### New Flavors

Do not overwhelm your baby with new tastes and experiences as the taste buds in an infant's mouth are not very developed and neither is the digestive system enough to take an onslaught of various solids. Introduce one flavor or solid at a time and give your baby a few days before introducing a new solid.

Though it is preferable that your baby be partial to all sorts of food and have a variety of intake, give your baby time to understand and come to terms with different textures and tastes so you can understand your baby's preferences. Generally, you should let the transition be from puree or liquefied foods to mashed food and then eventually to small pieces of food your baby can gum easily.

### Is My Baby Full?

Frequent growing, mood, and interest will vary your baby's appetite, so do not count on your baby's feeding frequencies to be an indication of your baby to be eating healthily. To know, however, that your baby is full, look for the following indicators:

- Turning head away from the food
- Leaning back
- Playing with something else and getting distracted
- Not opening mouth

### *Should I Put A Stop to Breast or Formula Milk?*

Absolutely not. Your baby requires the nutrients milk can only provide as the gradual transition to food does not meet the baby's need for vitamins, iron, and protein. It will take about a year for the baby to change his dependency on nutrition from milk to food.

### Tips on Solid Feedings:

Do not give food that could cause choking. Make sure the pieces are small and can be easily chewed since it could cause your baby to choke or puke.

Don't force your baby to try new food. Be patient and give new introductions time. If your baby is turning his or her head away from certain foods, it doesn't mean there is going to be a hard no in his or her life.

There's no order when it comes to taste, though your baby is born with a preference towards sweet food, it doesn't matter what order you divide or introduce sweets or savories in.

Poopy problems might occur since the introduction of solids is a new thing for the tiny intestines in your baby's tummy. The color, smell, and consistency of your baby's stool might change. Some doctors recommend giving your baby a fiber concentrated diet when constipation occurs, such as pears, apples, and prunes. It is still suggested that you see a doctor if your baby is having trouble passing stool or the bowel movements are taking far too much time to be released.

### How Many Feedings A Day?

When you start with the solids, your baby might not eat more than once a day but give it till your baby's 7th month and your baby will set the meal frequencies to two a day. Another month and it'll turn into three times a day.

A typical 8-month old's diet should consist of:

- Breast milk/formula milk
- Infant cereal
- Veggies
- Fruits
- Small amounts of protein such as dairy products, chicken, meat, and lentils

It is recommended that you not feed your baby honey until a year passes since it could cause botulism. Also, soy or cow milk should not be given until the first-year mark either.

### Homemade Baby Food

Some mothers like to make baby food themselves since it's always better to know what your baby is having. To make your own baby food, you'd need a blender or food grinder to make puree and storage containers so you can freeze the food if need be. For individual portions, you can use the ice tray.

It is also better that you get a convenient, heightened chair that is comfortable for your baby and prevents your baby from making the room look like a battlefield of a food fight. Make sure your baby is upright, so there's no swallowing hazard. Invest in a highchair once your baby can sit with stability. A highchair will help your baby be part of all family meals and it's much easier to clean up from a highchair than any other seating position.

### *Food Routine*

You must start introducing a routine when starting solids with your baby to form good habits that will continue and be helpful to the baby's health.

Make sure to wash the baby's hands, soothe him or her, and then sit him or her down to eat. Maintain calmness by turning the TV or loud music off to make the baby more aware of the food he or she is eating and recognizing when the tummy is full.

It might take some time for the baby to feel comfortable with the feel of spoons in the mouth and the different tastes and textures of the food.

Also, be prepared for a lot of mess. When solids are introduced, babies have more control of their hands, so be prepared for food to be flung everywhere. That doesn't mean your baby dislikes the food. It just means that your baby will be finding everything as a plaything.

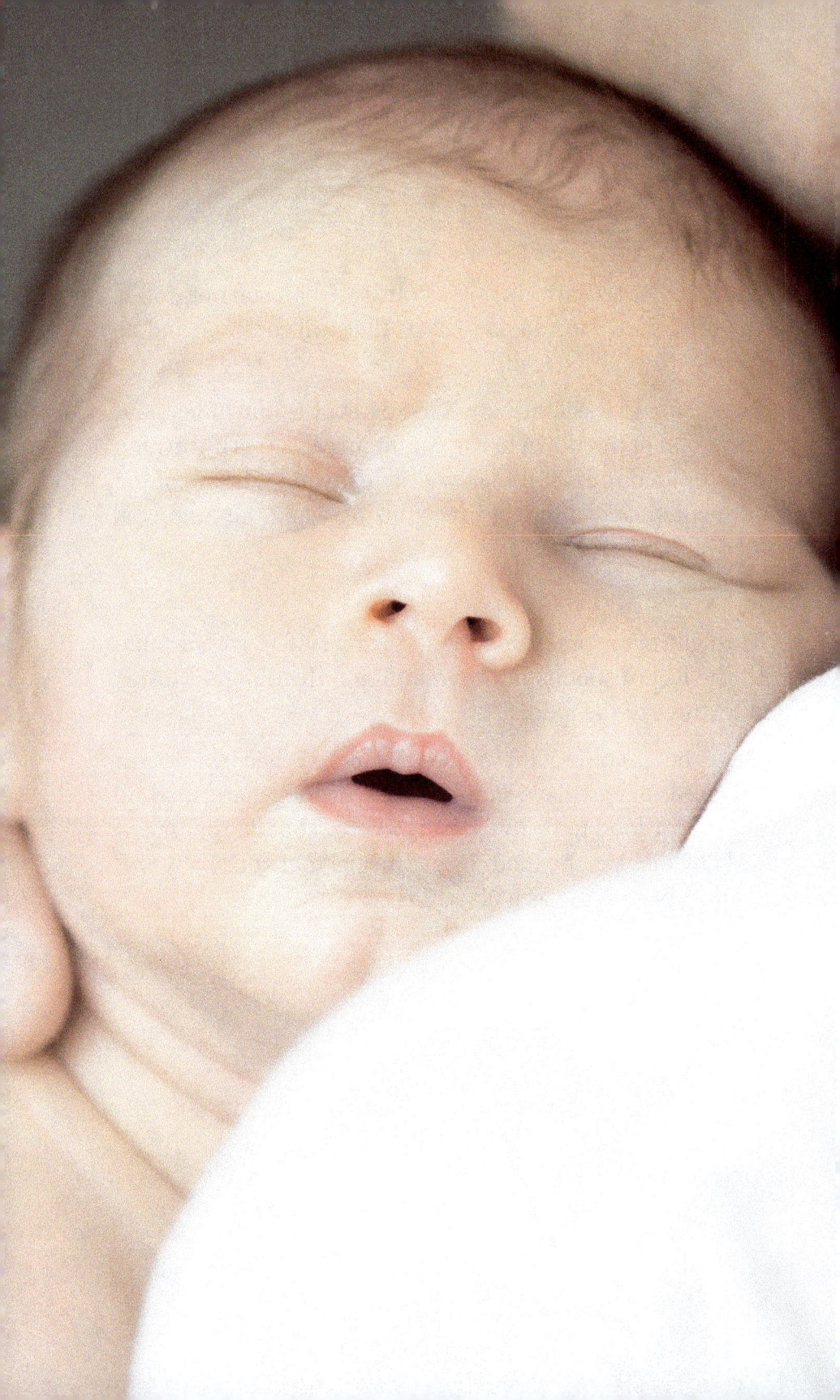

# Chapter 20: Mommy Brain and the Divider Mind

Not knowing what's going to happen in the next hour, day, or week is one of the most challenging parts of a high-risk pregnancy. The most natural reaction to such uncertainty when so much is at stake—when life is at stake—is to plan. You plan for worst-case scenarios. You make contingency plans. You make backup plans for backup plans. Whether those plans are just in your head or written down, or you act on them, the plans create some level of certainty, safety, and predictability.

They also create a false sense of relief and security.

While taking these preventative measures and preparing for the worst is smart and very practical, it doesn't alleviate the anxiety and worry you live with every day, wondering if you'll ever have to rely on these contingency plans. So, you double down on your efforts to make sure you don't need them.

You Google fervently to find stories of hope or information on how you can stay pregnant that your doctor may have forgotten to tell you. You analyze every symptom and try to understand where it's coming from. Was it a normal pain or was that a sign of something bad happening? You fight. All the time.

Who wouldn't? When your baby's life is on the line, what mother wouldn't fight with all her might all day, every day for as long as it takes?

That constant fight comes with a price.

Your physical and emotional stress is through the roof. You feel overwhelmed by each day, wondering how you're going to manage it all and stay sane.

Even worse is when it bleeds into your sleep, the "what ifs" getting louder as the house becomes quieter and darker. You might find it harder to fall back asleep too. Not only do you feel exhausted, but lack of sleep has been tied to many pregnancy complications such as preterm labor, premature rupture of membranes (water breaking too soon), and higher incidence of falling, 1 as well as placental abruption, 2 preeclampsia, 3 and preterm delivery, 4 so missing out on sleep is taking a physical toll on your body as well.

It might be scary to read all of this. I understand if you notice your heart racing a bit faster, your mouth feeling a bit dry, and starting to feel a bit jittery when you see how many factors play into the health of a pregnancy. I share this with you to also remind you that there is so much more in your control than you realize or are made to believe.

One way to achieve that is to give yourself permission to take a break from fighting all day, every day. You need it. Your body needs it. Even if you were being chased by a bear, you would find a place to hide and catch your breath, right? Similarly, during a high-risk pregnancy, you need to create that safe space where you feel comfortable stepping away from the fight for a few minutes or a few hours so your body can do what it does best when the self-repair system is on.

Your job is to give your body a chance to do just that. Where most women get stuck is not being able to turn off their brain. Many of them—and you may have done this, too—know they need to take a break. So, they lie down. Put their feet up. Turn on the TV. Go sit by the pool. They try their very best to relax. But their mind just keeps going. They're making lists in their head. Going over test results in their mind. Making their way through the long line of "what ifs." Unfortunately, just because your body isn't moving doesn't turn off the stress response in your body.5

Tap into your "inner pharmacy" by activating your relaxation response, and that allows your body the opportunity to do what it does best. This self-repair mechanism needs a chance to be activated regularly to help you stay pregnant for as long as possible. To do this requires you to take a break from the fight and the way to do that is to surrender to your reality.

I don't mean surrender as in "wave the white flag and give up." There's a stark difference between surrendering and giving up. Giving up means you stop trying. You walk away from the fight, throw your hands up, and believe there is absolutely nothing you can do to help yourself or your baby.

Surrendering is about reframing your pregnancy complications or situation by accepting the reality. This includes accepting what's happening, what's in your control, and what is not.

Surrendering is about deeply understanding that your body is not against you. It's about fully believing and trusting that, despite the health challenges you and your baby are facing, your body's number-one goal is to help you and your baby be healthy and safe. Your job is to believe that with every cell of your body and to give your body the opportunity to heal itself to the best of its ability (sometimes with the help of medical interventions) no matter what complications you are experiencing.

Surrendering is also about checking the thoughts that float in your head about yourself. Are you blaming yourself for these complications? Are you berating yourself for putting your baby's life in danger? Are you talking down to yourself for putting your career first and waiting so long to get pregnant? Are you telling yourself that you are not fit to be a mother, that you don't know what you're doing, that you are not good enough? Are you telling yourself you're worthy of help, support, and caring?

Most of my clients struggle with this. I did, too.

It's so easy to take the blame for your high-risk pregnancy and feel responsible for putting your baby and your family in this position and to feel like the only way through it is to fight. There's a very real fear women have that if they allow themselves to rest, that's when something bad will happen and they won't be prepared. In fact, resting and surrendering for a moment is exactly how you'll help yourself be prepared for whatever lies ahead.

It's mind-blowing how powerful your body is and what it's capable of even when you're in the middle of the biggest fight of your life. It takes my breath away every time I think of it and brings tears to my eyes every time, I see it happen for my clients.

One woman I worked with had been in and out of the hospital since she hit 20 weeks. She already had a history of preterm delivery and this pregnancy had shown signs of pregnancy complications even earlier than her previous one. Her doctor had warned her that she might deliver even earlier than her first and she should prepare herself for not making it too far into the third trimester.

After her third stint in the hospital, during which she described yelling at her partner and her mother-in-law purely out of stress, she reached out for help. She was fiercely determined to stay pregnant longer than her doctor was predicting and wanted to know what more she could do. Our work together, as with all my clients, was about allowing her body to heal and recover from the physical and emotional stress she was under. Not only did she never return to the hospital for an overnight visit, her preterm contractions became more infrequent, and when they did arise, she knew exactly how to stop them at home. Her blood pressure decreased, and she developed such confidence in her body that she would reassure her nurses not to worry because she knew what her body was capable of.

When you can tap into this "built-in pharmacy," you can fully experience how many tools we have at our disposal to help ourselves stay pregnant. Surrendering to your reality gives you a much-needed reprieve from the fight, which can tremendously improve your health during pregnancy. It's all about allowing your body to do what it is trying to do and what it does best: help you recover and heal from the impact of stress so you can stay pregnant.

Practicing mindfulness is one powerful tool to help you do just that and can be powerfully effective especially during pregnancy.6 I'll admit, this is a bit of a New Age buzzword right now, but it really does work. Mindfulness is "the practice of cultivating non-judgmental awareness in day-to-day life."7 But let's be honest, it's a huge concept that can feel overwhelming to take on when you have so much already weighing on you during your high-risk pregnancy.

My take on mindfulness, and how I teach it to my clients, is to get out of your head and into your body. Whether you're sitting at your desk at work, lying on the couch in the evening, or stuck in a hospital bed, your mind is likely swirling with thoughts that are strong, are powerful, and feel believable. Stopping those thoughts is important but the task can feel like trying to plug up a burst dam with a wine bottle cork.

My best advice: forget your thoughts and focus on your body.

This can be really challenging for most people. Almost every one of my clients finds this extremely powerful when they can do it, but at the beginning find it difficult. It's not their fault, nor yours. Most of us grow up very disconnected from our bodies. We get so caught up in our thoughts, trusting them as the ultimate truth, and handing over our bodies to medical professionals, medications, or alternative providers to fix when there's a problem. We look to a thermometer to tell us if we have a fever or a scale to tell us if we've gained or lost enough weight when our bodies are sharing this information with us all the time. This is one of the biggest reasons we miss the early warning signs.

Learning to listen to your body and be present in your body not only helps you through a health crisis like a high-risk pregnancy but is a life-long skill that will serve you in any situation that you find yourself going forward.

The easiest way to practice mindfulness by getting into your body is to put your hand on an object that is nearest to you. Maybe it's a pillow, a throw blanket, a water bottle, or even this book. Close your eyes and feel that object, describing it with as many words as you can. Try doing it for 30 seconds as this becomes easier, try for 60 seconds or longer.

A more advanced version of this exercise is to focus more deeply on your body and notice bodily sensations.

Do you have pain? Where is it? Describe it. Do you feel muscle tension? Where? How does it feel? Do you feel achy? Name the spots.

Focus also on positive sensations too. What parts of your body feel relaxed or comfortable? Or if you're having a particularly difficult day, which parts feel the least bad?

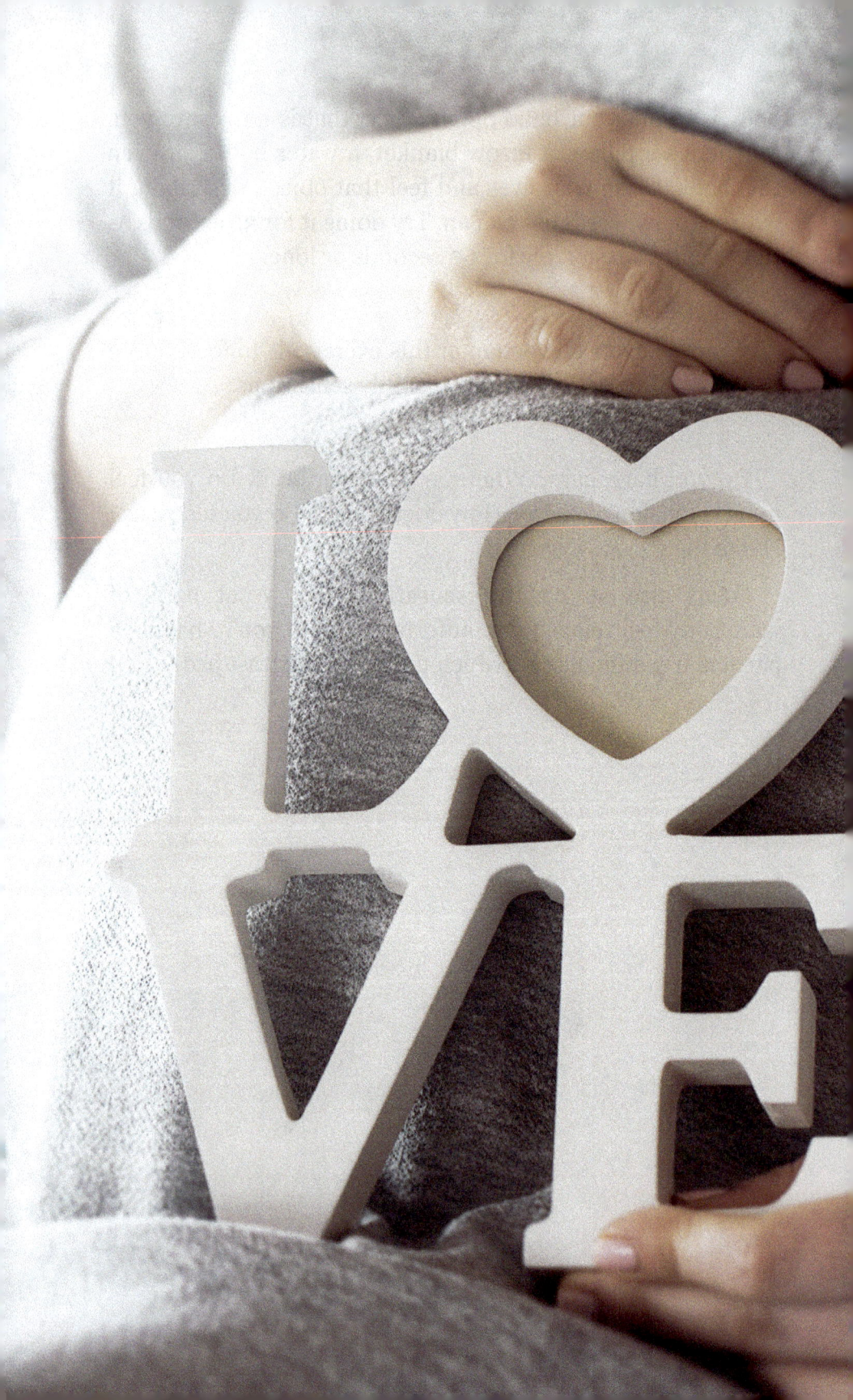

# Chapter 21: The Physical and Emotional Realities of Postpartum Sex

Sex will probably feel different. And at first, depending on hormones and healing, there may be some slight discomfort that requires generous lubrication and easing into intercourse with strategy, but sex should not hurt. Painful sex is never normal at any point in life. Don't settle for the advice that you should drink some wine, take a bath, and try to relax a little. Don't settle for the advice that you should just push through, and it will get better with time. There may be multiple physical and emotional components at play here.

• Physical elements: scar tissue, healing of muscles/tissue, hormones, tight muscles;

• Nervous system and emotional components: guarding of the body from trauma experienced during labor and birth, guarding against the previous time you've tried sex that became painful, and getting comfortable with your new body

If your body perceives that something will be painful, regardless of whether there is actual tissue damage, it will most likely be painful. This part will cover advice on how you can get comfortable with your vulva and vagina yourself and with your partner. Just like with returning to exercise, the progression you move through will be based on listening to your own body and what it's ready for. Consider seeking out help with a pelvic floor PT, postnatal specialists, and mental health/sex therapists to deal with the various components of your recovery. Also, consider lube!

Your vulva and vagina are most likely drier than they were before due to hormones, especially if you are breastfeeding. There are a lot of lubricant options out there, but my advice is to read the labels. Some lubricants that are well marketed can dry you out more or may have irritating additives and fragrances. Look for options without glycerin or parabens, no flavors, fragrances, or tingling effects. Opt for water-based or silicone-based lubricants (Slippery Stuff, Good Clean Love, Yes! Sliquid Organics, Uber Lube). Or consider coconut or olive oil from your kitchen cabinet but remember oil doesn't mix well with condoms.

«If pregnancy and childbirth weren't enough to put your pelvic floor through the wringer, breastfeeding is another event that affects your vagina. To keep your breast milk, source up, your estrogen points remain low. And low estrogen is pretty much like your vagina is in menopause, which is why your vagina feels similar to a desert throughout sex and your period does not come back until breastfeeding decreases.

Low estrogen implies your vaginal tissues are dried up, thin, and not as reassuring until your estrogen levels improve as your baby grows older and needs less and less breastmilk. Pelvic floor PT can also help progress circulation to your pelvic floor, bid tips for vaginal drought, and aid your muscles to stay solid to prevent seepage and prolapse, as your vagina is still in the recovery phase while breastfeeding. So, mommas, be patient, be kind to your vagina, and be proactive in its strengthening and healing phase by working with a pelvic floor PT during postpartum recovery.»

—Sara Reardon, PT, DPT, WCS, BCB-PMD

### How can You Ease Back to Intimacy?

Here are some examples of how you can ease back into intimacy with your partner. Choose ways that feel comfortable and appropriate for your goals. Often, our lack of awareness, comfort, and confidence in knowing this part of our body may contribute to fear, pain, and tension we feel.

### Feeling yourself

1. Next time you're in the shower or have some time to lie down in a relaxed position, start by feeling your abdominal and pelvic region. Simply begin with the goal of feeling the tissues and muscles on the outside. If you had a cesarean birth, start to feel your lower abdomen and work on making peace with touching this area. For some this may be easy. For others, it's extremely triggering. The next part will cover scar tissue in more detail. If you're not ready to touch your scars yet, skip this part. Feel around the rest of your belly. Feel the skin, the muscles, the stretch marks. Get comfortable with your own hands touching your body. Move on to your pelvic area. Touch your vulva. Feel the labia majora and the labia minora and the clitoris. Feel your way around externally and see if there are any painful areas. If so, work on gentle touching that area in a way that does not cause pain. Use gentle touch in a slow, intentional way to increase your positive experience in self-exploration rather than pushing through pain.

2. Progress by starting to feel internally. Do so gently. Pretend your vaginal opening is a clock with 12:00 being up towards the urethra/clitoris and 6:00 being towards the anus. Begin by slowly inserting one finger into your vagina towards the 6:00 position. Hold there for a bit and simply sense how it feels. Slowly move your finger towards the 3:00 position, then

back to the 6:00, and then toward the 9:00 position. Take your time and try to make this a positive or at least neutral experience. Do not push into pain. Take full breaths as you're doing this and think positive thoughts.

3. Advance to feel deeper and/or with more speed. Continue to feel in different directions and depths of your vagina. Use different pressures. Feel your pelvic floor muscles internally: contract, relax, and lengthen. Feel your breath gently expand and contract these muscles at a low level naturally. Notice if there are any areas that feel tight or painful and slowly work to bring gentle touch and release to those areas.

4. Continue to touch and feel internally and externally in any way that you may encounter during sexual intercourse. Use this time to make peace with your body and experience physically and mentally. Note if there are certain areas that you will want to be careful and mindful of while returning to intercourse with your partner. Only pursue this exercise as a positive, pain-free experience. Another way some women find helpful to advance at this point is using a dilator, wand, or sex toys at this point as progression to partner intimacy. Vibration has been shown to help with healing tissue and scars.

### Sex and Other Forms of Intimacy

When you feel ready and want to begin being intimate with your partner, have an open conversation about going slowly and speaking up if something doesn't feel right. You may not jump right back into positions or speeds you were used to previously. There may be different positions that are less painful and allow you to feel more in control of the depth of penetration. There are lots of options as you heal physically and emotionally. As hormones settle back down and you work through the above steps, you should be able to return to sex pain-free.

The same way you've worked through touching yourself slowly and intentionally may be something you want to work through with your partner. You may choose to start with external stimulation rather than any forms of penetration if that feels right for you. The more open and honest you can be your partner can help you into making this a positive, pain-free activity you'll continue to enjoy in the long run.

Don't put pressure on yourself to orgasm right away. Find ways to reach the orgasm externally with the clitoris rather than pushing through anything (friction, speed, positions, length of time) you're not ready for it internally.

Again, you should not push through the pain. There are specific ways a pelvic floor PT can help you postpartum to work through the physical things at play. A PT can help you better understand how the nervous system and brain is responding in a protective way and how to work through that. Considering talking with a medical provider about hormone contribution if these methods are not helping dryness.

Every woman will get back to sex at different rates based on healing, hormones, and sex drive. Give yourself time and grace to connect with your pelvic floor muscles, breath, vulva, vagina, clitoris, and abdomen. You are beautiful and resilient. You've got this!

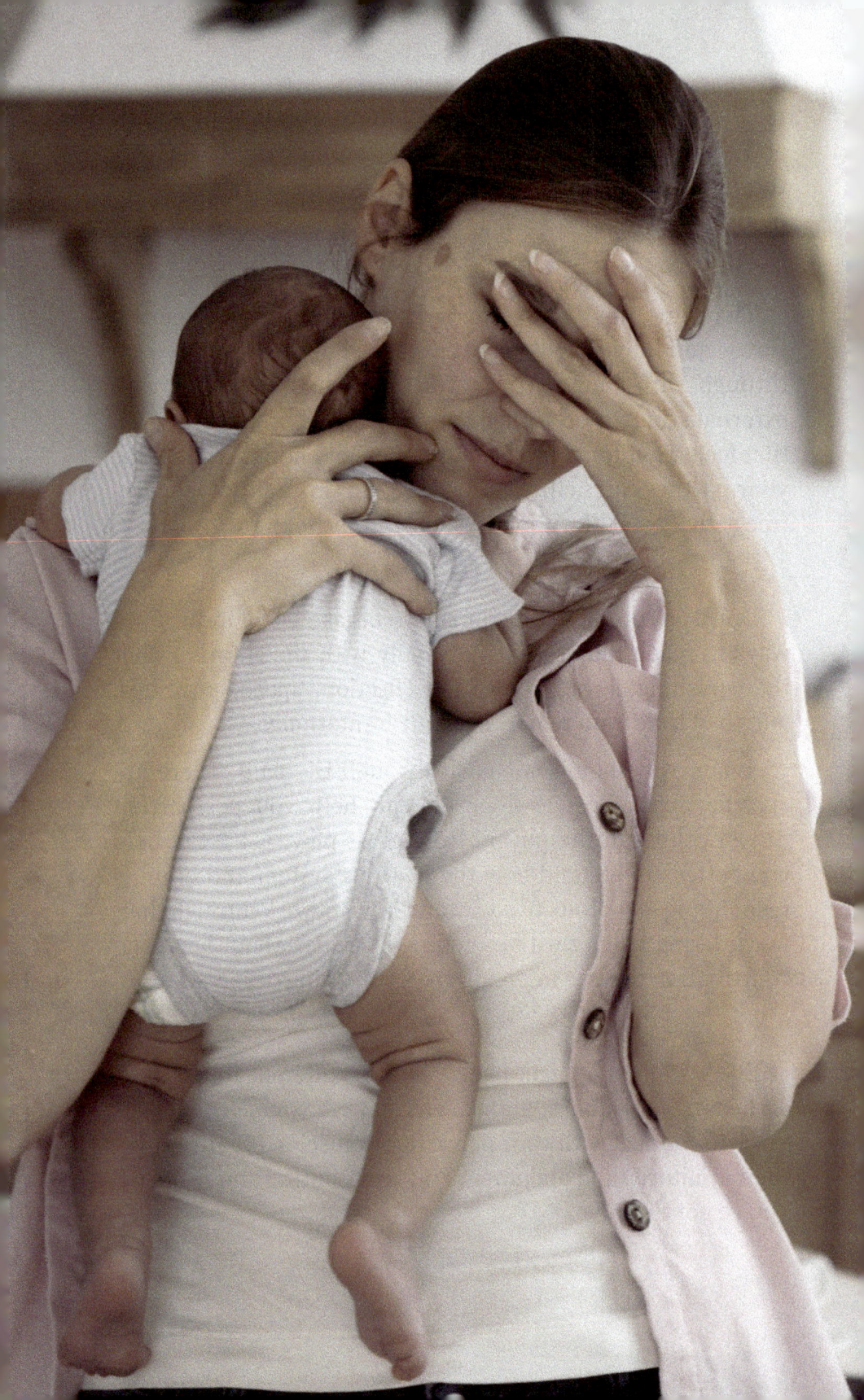

# Chapter 22: The Baby Blues Versus Postpartum Depression Versus Postpartum Anxiety

### *Postpartum Depression*

As a new mother, you only hear about the joys of motherhood. You hear about what it feels like to meet your baby for the first time, the bond that you have. What happens when your experience is not like this at all? Maybe you deliver your baby, only to realize that you are very depressed, not connected to anyone. If this happens to you, know that this is a normal condition experienced by many mothers worldwide. This is postpartum depression, and it is a common condition for new moms to develop. No matter how much you have been looking forward to having your baby, the postpartum depression can still rise to the surface before you realize what is happening.

There is not only a single reason why you might develop the condition, but there are a few prominent factors. Hormones can have something to do with it. After you give birth, your estrogen levels and progesterone levels experience a big drop. When you have been living with elevated levels for nearly a year, your body gets used to this. As these hormones drop, your thyroid function can also drop. This is what leaves you feeling depressed and sluggish. Changes in your blood pressure, immune system, and metabolism can all trigger your experience with postpartum depression, as well.

### What is the Difference Between PPD and Baby Blues?

A common condition that mothers develop after pregnancy is the baby blues. This differs from postpartum depression (PPD) because it is not as serious. Immediately after childbirth, it is common for the new mother to experience at least a bit of baby blues. This has something to do with the sudden change in hormones in your body, but it can also be combined with the stress experienced during delivery. After giving birth, everything seems to be moving very quickly for you and your new baby, causing you to feel overwhelmed and fatigued. Don't worry because this is bound to change very soon. Once you get used to your routine, you will usually be able to beat the baby blues.

When you have the baby blues, you might feel extra emotional in the days to follow your delivery. This can mean more tearful moments and more emotional fragility. Know that this is perfectly normal. You will notice a peak in these symptoms after one week postpartum, but then you can expect them to taper off by the time that you enter the second week. This is a good indication that what you are experiencing is the baby blues. It should not last much longer than this. If it does, you might need to consult your doctor to determine if you are suffering from PPD.

You can think of the baby blues as mild depression, whereas PPD is more severe depression. When you have mild depression, mood swings are still common. One moment, you might be happy to be spending time with your baby and your family, and then that feeling will subside and become replaced with stress or anxiety. This is new for you, so don't forget to give yourself plenty of time to breathe. Needing a break does not make you a bad or weak mom. Ensure that your partner plays an equal role to prevent either one of you from feeling burnt out. Your partner can help you a lot during times when you feel that you have the baby blues. By picking up the slack, you won't be left feeling quite so overwhelmed.

### *What Are Recognizable Symptoms?*

PPD is something that should not go ignored. Because it is a more intense form of depression than the baby blues, you might need to consult your doctor for a solution. When you have PPD, you will experience a wide range of symptoms. Pay attention to the severity of each symptom that you feel and see if you can relate to these. Some of the most common symptoms are the following:

- **Withdrawing:**

After giving birth, you probably imagined that you would feel closer to your new family than ever. Every moment leading up to the delivery showed you that you would be spending plenty of time enjoying your baby and bonding with your partner over the new arrival. You might be experiencing symptoms of withdrawal if things do not go as planned.

No matter who you are withdrawing from, your baby or partner, this is a sign that PPD might be occurring. If you feel that you cannot bond with your baby or are no longer close with your partner, know that this feeling will pass with the proper treatment.

- **Anxiety:**

When you have anxiety that is out of control, it will impact you mentally and physically. You might not be able to eat or sleep, which makes it much more difficult to take care of

157

your baby. To provide them with nourishment, you need to be taking the best care of yourself. Your mind will run wild with the what-ifs, torturing you into thinking that you aren't doing a good job.

Even when your baby appears fine, like eating or sleeping, you might be second-guessing yourself and wondering why you are doing everything wrong. This type of anxiety can place a lot of unrealistic expectations on you, preventing you from enjoying this time that you have with your newborn.

- **Guilt:**

You might experience feeling washed over by guilt after you give birth to your baby. You might feel guilty over how you delivered your baby or how much you can give them now that they are born. These thoughts will keep cycling through your mind, making you preoccupied.

When you have intense guilt, this can make even the most enjoyable moments stressful because you are constantly worrying. It is easy to move past the guilt and focus on the positive sides, but PPD makes this part difficult. This might prove to be a feeling that you cannot shake.

- **Worthlessness:**

It can be very hard to experience worthlessness when you have a new baby to care for. They depend on you for everything, from nourishment to shelter. On the inside, all you might be able to feel is that your life no longer matters. On some days, you might even wish that you could just disappear altogether.

- **Suicidal Thoughts:**

One of the most serious symptoms of PPD is suicidal

thoughts. Just because you have PPD does not automatically mean that you will develop these thoughts, but you must look out for them. Becoming preoccupied with death, or wanting to die, is very dangerous and should be reported to a medical professional. If you are experiencing this, do not delay telling someone and getting help.

The sooner you open to someone you trust, the sooner you will feel relief from your PPD symptoms. Motherhood is not all stress and worry. You can enjoy your life in your new role. Lean on your partner for extra support when necessary. Look at your baby, remembering that you brought them into this world. You completed a huge task already, and you are wonderful for doing so.

### *Best Coping Strategies*

There are ways to cope with your PPD, no matter how severe it gets. When you prioritize taking care of your baby, this automatically means that you must take care of yourself. What you can provide for your baby is a direct extension of what you can provide for yourself. While this time is going to be difficult for you, know that this is not what it will feel like forever.

- Create a Secure Attachment:

Known as an attachment, this is the emotional bonding process that occurs between you and your baby. To create a secure attachment, you must pay attention to your baby. When they are feeling discomfort, try to soothe them right away. After they start crying, offer them solutions, whether they are cuddles or feeding.

Your baby is going to feel secure when they know that you are always there for them. It is a way to build trust that your baby will understand, even as an infant. This is how you will set yourself up for a great relationship with your baby as they grow older. It will also show you that you have plenty of purpose and reason to be there, as PPD can often trick you into feeling otherwise.

- Lean on Others for Help:

You don't have to keep your feelings to yourself. If you don't want to admit exactly how you feel to your partner, consider opening to another mother. You would be surprised at how many other mothers have also dealt with PPD and successfully overcame it.

Even if you don't want to go very in-depth, it helps to have emotional support. Anyone who appears supportive in your life right now should be someone you are spending time with. Don't forget to prioritize these relationships in your life.

- Take Care of Yourself:

After giving birth, you shouldn't have to jump back into doing all the housework. Let your partner take care of this, as you need to take care of your body. While the first thing you might want to do is make the house as perfect as possible, put yourself first. Make sure that you are fully healed before you get back into any kind of physical activity.

When you do start feeling better in a few weeks, you can get back into low-impact exercise. This involves walking and doing gentle at-home workouts. The endorphin rush will help you combat your PPD. By exercising, you will also be getting better sleep at night. This is essential for any new parent and practices some mindfulness meditation to clear your head.

- Make Time for Your Partner:

Your partner has now been filled with ways to take care of your infant—this is natural, but you don't want to let your little one takes over every opportunity you get with your partner. Keep your relationship strong during this time. You will both need mutual support.

When your baby is asleep, check-in with your partner, see how they are doing and what they are feeling. You both know the experience best, as you are raising the same child. Don't forget to engage in intimate moments together. Even if you don't feel like having sex yet, cuddling, kissing, and hugging is a great way to re-enter the intimacy.

- Seek Professional Help:

If you feel that you cannot handle your PPD on your own, commend yourself by taking the big step. Your doctor will be able to help you in a few ways. One of which is attending individual therapy or marriage counseling. Talking to a professional can be enough to ease your mind. When you can get the worrisome things off your chest, you are making more room for happiness.

Antidepressants or hormone therapy might also be recommended to you. No matter which is recommended, your doctor will be keeping a close eye on you to make sure that you are reacting well to the medication and that you are safe.

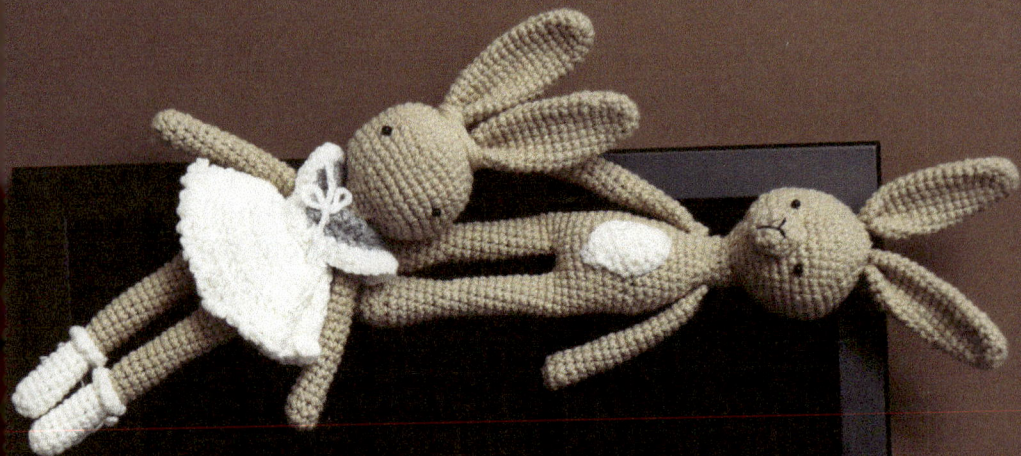

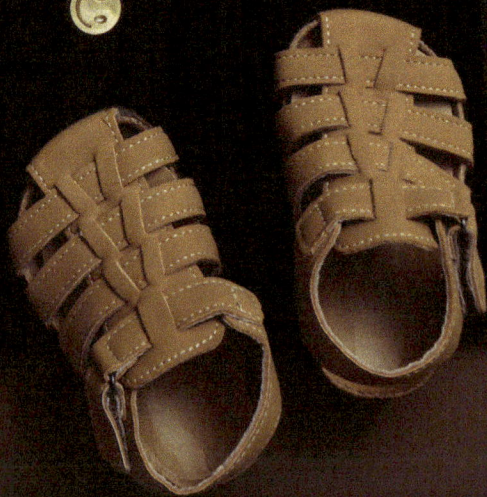

# Chapter 23: Baby Blues

Many women face the postpartum depression. This problem is known as "baby blues" and hits all groups of women – first-time moms and moms who already had a baby. Even dads can be affected by postpartum depression.

No matter if you wanted your baby so badly, and couldn't wait to meet her in person, sometimes you can feel down and depressed after the delivery. You always need to remember that feeling sadness does not make you a bad mother – you just went through a life changing experience. Your body and brain are still full of hormones that affect your health.

Feeling depressed can be confusing and upsetting – you actually thought you would feel joy and happiness, but yet, you start crying for no reason, you are worried all the time, feel tiredness and have self-doubt.

While "baby blues" often passes within a week or two, sometimes it can last a little longer. It is a normal thing to ask for help and support from your partner, parents, and friends. You shouldn't keep your emotions to yourself – if you want to cry, you should cry – it will make you feel better later. You should always keep in mind that you went through the stressful event and you have a new situation that you need to get used to it. You can have troubles with sleeping, identity crises, concerns about parenthood and caring for a newborn child, feeling of loss of control over life and other similar feelings.

Congratulations, you now have a baby! After reading this book, you should now have a good grasp of what you expect throughout your pregnancy as well as how your baby is going to grow and change.

From the time you ovulate until the time you have your baby in your arms, your body is going to undergo immense changes. Your baby is going to change from a tiny cell that isn't visible to the naked eye to an almost eight-pound being that is going to fill your life and heart with joy.

What is important to point out is that you should carefully monitor your condition. If you feel unusually intense, having suicide thoughts, or can't do your simple daily tasks, like taking care of your hygiene, you should ask for help from your doctor and seek treatment. The doctor can advise you counseling or prescribe antidepressant medication (or both). Getting the right treatment is very important. What you should know is that you are not alone – a lot of woman goes through the same thing. The most important thing to know is that, with the right treatment, postpartum depression can be successfully healed.

# Chapter 24: Care for Postpartum Depression and Baby Blues

During pregnancy, birth, and post-delivery a woman's body goes through countless physical and hormonal changes. Because of this, it is normal to have a period where all your hormones haven't quite yet balanced. This period can take place anywhere from a few days after birth to 6 months postpartum. Every woman's body is different and how it adjusts and heals is different. This period also coincides with the growing pains that having a new baby in the house brings to every family.

Women are getting less sleep than normal as they are up multiple times throughout the night for feedings. This is a very difficult adjustment period for many women. Often during this time of adjustment, a woman can become weepy and feel down. This feeling is known as the baby blues. It is important that we clarify that there is a difference between a minor case of the baby blues and true postpartum depression.

Postpartum depression should be treated by your doctor because it can be very serious. In this portion, we are going to deal with a mild case of the baby blued and natural ways that you can deal with these feelings.

It is important to remember that your body has just undergone many extreme changes in a very short period. You are physically still healing from the ordeal of labor and delivery. You are also adjusting to a new family dynamic and getting less sleep than normal. Remember to give yourself grace and not to expect too much of yourself, too soon. It will take time for you to heal, get used to your new life with your baby and to start to get a handle on regular life. Don't expect it all to happen overnight. It is a process that requires rest, healing, good nutrition, and help from your family and friends.

- Relax and rest. - The first few months with a newborn are exhausting. You will need to put aside all other commitments and just focus on your baby and healing. The most important thing you can do is to sleep when your baby sleeps. Newborns are on very different schedules than the rest of the world. They need to eat every few hours. You will not be getting long uninterrupted periods of sleep. So, sleep when your baby is sleeping. If you are unable to sleep then relax during that time. Do not try to clean the house or make a big meal. Instead, take that time for your body and mind to rest and heal.

- Keep your baby close. - For the first few months after your baby is born, it is a good idea to keep your baby in your room, close to your bed. This will allow for easier middle of the night feedings and both baby and mom will get more rest.

- Don't over socialize- Family and friends will all be excited to meet your new bundle of joy but do not feel pressured into having too many visitors. Take this time to bond with your baby and to heal your body. You do what you feel comfortable and able to do, no more. Do not feel guilty for setting healthy boundaries for you and your baby.

• Take a walk. - Go outside and get a bit of fresh air every day. This is good for you both physically and mentally. Take a short walk if you can. This will help you to improve your mood and to feel better physically.

• Eat- Your body is not only recovering from being pregnant, labor and delivery, you are also feeding another human from it if you are nursing. For your body to be able to do all these things, you need to eat a balanced and nutritious diet. Lactation specialist recommends that eat when you feel hungry. However, many new moms are too exhausted to eat when they have a chance to or are focused on losing the baby weight and skip meals. Skipping meals will inhibit weight loss as it puts your body into starvation mode. You will lose muscle not fat. It is very important to eat a balanced and nutrient-packed diet. In the next portion, we will explore what a healthy diet for a nursing mom looks like.

### Postpartum Nutrition

An easy way to be sure that you are getting proper nutrition is to follow the USDA MyPlate nutrition program. MyPlate is a visual representation of what the proper portion sizes of the five main food groups are.

### The Five Food Groups

**Grains**: Thirty percent of your plate should be made up of food from the grain's category. It is best to eat whole grain foods rather than highly processed grains like white bread. Grains consist of foods such as wheat, rice, cornmeal, oats, and quinoa. Pasta, breads, and porridges are considered grains.

**Vegetables**:  Forty percent of your plate should be made up of foods from the vegetable category.  There is a large assortment of vegetables from which you can choose.  A good basic rule of thumb is that the more colorful the vegetable the better it is for you.  For instance, orange sweet potatoes and yams are healthier for you than white potatoes are.  Make your plate as colorful as possible.

**Fruit**:  Ten percent of your plate should be made up of fruit.  You can eat any fruit that you like.  Fruits are full of antioxidants and vitamins and are very healthy for you.

**Protein**:  Twenty percent of your plate should be made up of a protein.  Proteins are meat, fish, eggs, beans, and nuts.  Protein is particularly important as you heal from your labor and delivery and while you are nursing.

**Dairy**:  Dairy should be a 4-8 oz serving for a normal diet but if you are nursing you will require more dairy.  Dairy consist of foods such as milk, cheese, and yogurt.

**Oils**:  Although oils are not an official part of the USDA MyPlate program, there are some very beneficial oils for new moms.  Coconut oil, olive oil, some nut oils are all good nutrition while nursing.  You should avoid saturated fats and solid animal fats like butter or lard.

If possible, eat organic foods that have not been processed.  These will have a higher nutritional value and will be healthier for you and your baby.

### Exercise

It is important to include some sort of physical exercise into your daily routine once your body is healed enough. This is good for your mental health as well as your physical wellbeing. A simple daily walk for thirty minutes outside will do wonders for you. If you want to get back into a more intense exercise regimen wait to be cleared by your doctor or midwife and then you are free to work back into your normal exercise regimen.

Most women are concerned about losing those extra baby pounds. It can take a little bit of time to lose those stubborn pounds but don't be discouraged. You just grew an entire person in your body. It is normal to need a minute to bounce back from that. Starving yourself and skipping meals is the worst way to lose weight. If you are nursing, you can also harm your baby by not getting enough calories and nutrition. Eating a healthy balanced diet with moderate exercise is the best way to lose that baby weight.

It is very important to stay well hydrated while you are nursing. You will dehydrate much more quickly. Make sure you drink plenty of water and milk.

### Help from Family and Friends

During the first few weeks to months, it is very beneficial for new parents to have help from family and friends. This is particularly important for mom to get the rest she needs and for her mental health. Having a family member or friend help with some of the household chores and with some of the baby care so that both parents can rest and maybe grab a quick shower is an amazing gift. A good support network is one of the largest contributing factors towards a new mother's good mental health. On the flip side, studies have shown new mothers with little or no support network are much more likely to develop postpartum depression. Having clear communication with the family and friends that are helping is important to avoid any misunderstandings. Be clear with your needs and express gratitude for their help but do not feel pressured into doing things their way instead of what works for you and your infant.

### *Breathing Strategies*

- Breath Counting- Take a deep breath in through your nose. Count as you are breathing in...2...3...4. Now breathe out through your mouth. Count as you breathe out, your breath out should be a bit longer than your breath in. Breathe out...2...3...4...5...6. While breathing keep your shoulders back and your jaw relaxed.


- Visualization- Close your eyes and try to think of a color that relaxes you. Pick the first relaxing color that comes to your mind. Keep your eyes closed and focus on that color. Think about how vibrant it is and why you find it relaxing. Now visualize breathing this color in through your nose. Take a deep breath and fill your lungs with this color. Feel the color move down through your abdomen into your womb. Once in your womb, it swirls around your baby bringing them comfort and relaxation. Now breathe the color out through your slightly open mouth. Watch the color as it drifts away, taking away all your stress and tension. Do this visualization exercise in sets of three repetitions.


- Mantras- Mantras are repeated words or sounds that

help you to relax and focus. They can put you in touch with the rhythms of your body and mind. You can make up your own mantra or you can use one that is already created. Here is an example: As you deeply breathe in and exhale slowly and completely repeat these phrases "I inhale rest. I exhale exhaustion." "I inhale calm. I exhale tension." "I inhale strength and exhale weakness." "I inhale love and exhale negativity." Repeat this set of mantras three times. End by taking a deep breath in and slowly blowing an exhaling breath. Keep your muscles loose and relax.

Practice these breathing techniques at the end of the day, every day, for several months before labor and delivery. Keep your eyes closed and try to focus inwardly. Allow yourself to completely relax while doing these breathing exercises.

### Positive Affirmations for Labor and Delivery

Repeat these affirmations several times a day, every day, in the months preparing for labor and delivery.

- I will have a quick and safe delivery.

- My birthing experience will go smoothly and be painless. I think I can and therefore I will.

- Every contraction and push bring my baby closer to me.

- Women around the world are delivering their babies while I deliver mine.

- Breathing slowly and deeply relaxes my muscles making my labor much easier.

- I am strong.

- I trust my body to know how to birth my baby just as it knew how to grow my baby.

- I breathe deeply through each contraction, giving both my body and my baby the oxygen, they need.

- I stay active and healthy so that my baby will be born on time, without complications.

# Chapter 25: What Happens to Your Body After Delivery?

After either a vaginal birth or caesarean section the body and mind changes

## Lochia

After birthing your body will be getting rid of mucus, blood, and tissue debris. For 3 to 5 days, blood loss will be bright red and heavier than a normal period. You may also pass clots. It becomes pinker between day 5 and 9 then brown and eventually yellow-white. The bleeding may stop after 2 to 3 weeks or go on for up to 6 weeks after birth.

You may need to change the pad every hour or two at the beginning and every 3 to 4 hours later.

Watch out for signs of infection. If you experience an unpleasant smell, have a fever, the bleeding is still bright red and heavy following the first week or your belly feels sore low down on one or both sides go to see your GP.

## Baby blues

Over half of new mothers experience the baby blues. It usually happens 3 or 4 days after the birth and is an indication that milk is coming in. Hormones are all over the place and you may find yourself crying inconsolably for no reason. You may also experience an anti-climax, exhaustion, feel overwhelmed at being a mother or have feelings of grief for losing your bump. It may last from a few hours to a few days. For a smaller number of mothers, the baby blues might only kick in after a couple of weeks and therefore catch them unawares.

Going through the baby blues does not mean you suffer from post-natal depression (see Postpartum health red flags). Be kind to yourself. You have just gone through enormous physical and emotional changes. Use your support network to its maximum and try and rest as much as possible. The "fog" will soon lift.

## Pain

If you are in pain, make sure you take adequate pain relief. Tell your midwife or GP if your pain is not controlled.

You may want to use a pillbox with 4 daily compartments to ensure you take pain killers at regular intervals. It is recommended to take pain medication before the pain worsens to keep on top of it.

### Afterpains

As your uterus contracts back after birth, afterpains are to be expected. They feel like period or stomach cramps and range from mild to severe. They sometimes ramp up when you breastfeed. These will stop after a few weeks.

### Back Pain

Back pain is common during pregnancy and can carry on after birth or develop postpartum.

Conservative treatment is recommended:

• Keep pelvic floor and core muscles active by sitting, standing, and walking tall

• Start pelvic floor exercises as soon as possible

• Avoid lifting heavy objects (a baby car seat for example) until your pelvic floor muscles are stronger

• When you can lift heavy objects again, bend your knees, keep your back straight and hold the object close to your body. Brace by squeezing your pelvic floor then deep stomach muscles before you start lifting. Use your thigh muscles as you lift.

• Kneel and squat to do low-level jobs such as bathing your baby

• Support your lower back with a cushion or pillow when you feed or when you drive

• Keep your back straight when you push your buggy or pram

• Use a changing table to change nappies

• Use heat packs and massage to relief tight spinal and buttock muscles

## Hemorrhoids (Piles) And Anal Fissures

You are more likely to suffer from these conditions if your baby was big, if labour was prolonged and/or birth caused significant injuries such as a severe tear, if your baby was delivered by forceps, if constipation is not dealt with and becomes chronic. Hemorrhoids are more common than anal fissures after birth. Around 10% of new mothers suffer from anal fissure.

These conditions should heal within a week or two, but they can be very painful and therefore require attention

- Use stool softeners, eat a high fiber diet, and drink plenty of water. Avoid constipation at all cost

- Don't push nor strain when you empty your bowels. This will worsen the problem

- Use wet wipes instead of toilet paper to clean and soothe the area

- Continue daily pelvic floor exercises and avoid heavy lifting

- Ask your midwife or your GP which ointment would be best to relieve swelling, inflammation, pain, and itching

## Changes to Your Skin

Stretch marks appear in pregnancy. You may find them on your tummy, bottom, thighs, and breasts. Sadly, you cannot get rid of stretch marks. However, they will fade over time and the streaks will blend more with your own skin color.

If you developed melasma during pregnancy, keep using sunblock. Most cases resolve spontaneously within a year following pregnancy. For a small number of women some dark patches persist, and you may need year-round sun protection. Some contraceptive pills may make the problem worse. Talk to your GP to decide which form of contraception suits you best.

If you have a linea nigra on your belly, it will fade away within a few weeks after birth.

## Hot Flushes and Night Sweats

This is very common after giving birth. Hot flushes and

night sweats can start a few days after delivery and can last for up to 6 weeks. In most cases, they subside after 7 to 8 days.

## Breasts

In the days following birth, your breasts will produce colostrum and should feel soft. When they start making milk, they will feel hot, swollen, and tender maybe even painful and this can last from a day to a fortnight. If you are breastfeeding put your baby at the breast as soon and as often as possible after birth so she can start learning how to feed when your breasts are soft. If your breasts are engorged, use hot compresses, or take a hot shower before a feed.

If breastfeeding, your nipples will be very sensitive. The beginning of each feed might feel uncomfortable. Even though unpleasant this is all quite normal. Your skin is getting used to your baby latching on. Apply nipple cream after each feed to create a moisture barrier and help keep your skin intact. If after 5 to 10 days you still experience problems such as cracked nipples or even bleeding, ask for help. A breastfeeding counsellor is the best person to call.

Once you stop breastfeeding, your breasts will return to how they were. The effects of pregnancy (rather than a consequence of breastfeeding) may make them a little less perky and not quite as self-supporting as before. If you are using formula, your breasts will stop producing milk and it may take a few months for them to return to their regular size.

## Swollen Feet and Hands

The extra fluid retained during pregnancy should start decreasing within a week or two of giving birth. If the swelling is persistent or painful, talk to your GP.

### Varicose Veins

Pregnancy is a risk factor for developing varicose veins. Sometimes they may develop in the pelvic area. In many cases, varicose veins significantly improve after birth and no treatment is required. Talk to your GP if you have any concerns.

### Hair Loss

Pregnancy hormones will have prevented your normal hair loss and you might have noticed you had thicker, more luxuriant hair. As soon as the hormone levels drop after birth, you may start losing a lot of hair. Don't panic. This is not glamorous, but your hair will eventually return to what it was.

### Return to exercise

Return to exercise should be gentle and gradual. Listen to your body. Women recover at different rates and only you will be able to feel what you can and can't do yet.

Reclaiming a strong body must start with exercising the pelvic floor muscles. In the first few weeks after birth, focus on re-establishing a daily routine of pelvic floor exercises and walking, sitting, and standing tall. Strengthening pelvic floor and core muscles must come before any other type of exercise.

To exercise the pelvic floor muscles, follow the routine given at the beginning of the book (see Basic health advice, Pelvic floor exercises).

To work on your deep abdominal muscles (or "core") follow this routine.

### Abdominal hollowing exercise

1.  Lie down on your back or on your side with your knees bent or sit with your back well supported

2.  Place your hands below your belly button

3.  Breathe in through your nose and as you breathe out to draw in your lower abdomen towards your back

4.  Relax

Start with a few repetitions and gradually increase the number of repetitions, holding the muscle drawn in for up to 10 seconds. Repeat 3 times a day if you can.

Once your core muscles are a little stronger, practice this exercise standing (before lifting or when changing baby for example).

Taking up exercise again will depend on how straight forward labour and birth were, your general fitness level, how quickly your pelvic floor and core muscles are strengthening, your exercise history and how easy it is for you to organize your time.

### Things to avoid

• Until you have had your postnatal check and you have stopped bleeding for a week, avoid swimming. This is to prevent infection.

• For up to 6 months after birth, pregnancy hormones will affect your joints. It is recommended you avoid vigorous and high impact exercise such as running, aerobics or sit-ups. Your pelvic floor and core muscles also need to be strong before resuming this type of exercise.

## A possible timeframe to resume exercise

Birth to 3 months

- Re-establish a daily routine of pelvic floor exercises
- Walk, stand, and sit tall
- Gentle core exercises

After your 6-week check or when your GP has given you all-clear

- Easy swimming
- Buggy fit classes
- Postpartum exercise classes (clinical Pilates for example)
- Low impact activities: swimming, aqua aerobics, basic belly dancing, tai chi

Between 3 and 6 months, providing you are not experiencing any problems and you have strengthened your pelvic and core muscles

- Pilates, yoga
- Activities you had before pregnancy

Returning to more challenging exercise should be delayed for 6 to 12 months in the following situations: you had a c-section, you sustained a serious injury (third and fourth degree tears), you had a prolonged second stage of labour with an instrumental delivery, you had a postpartum infection, you needed further surgery, if pelvic girdle pain is ongoing, you have been diagnosed with diastasis recti, you suffer from coccyx pain, you have a pelvic organ prolapse and/or suffer from incontinence. In some cases, it might be recommended you avoid high impact exercise indefinitely.

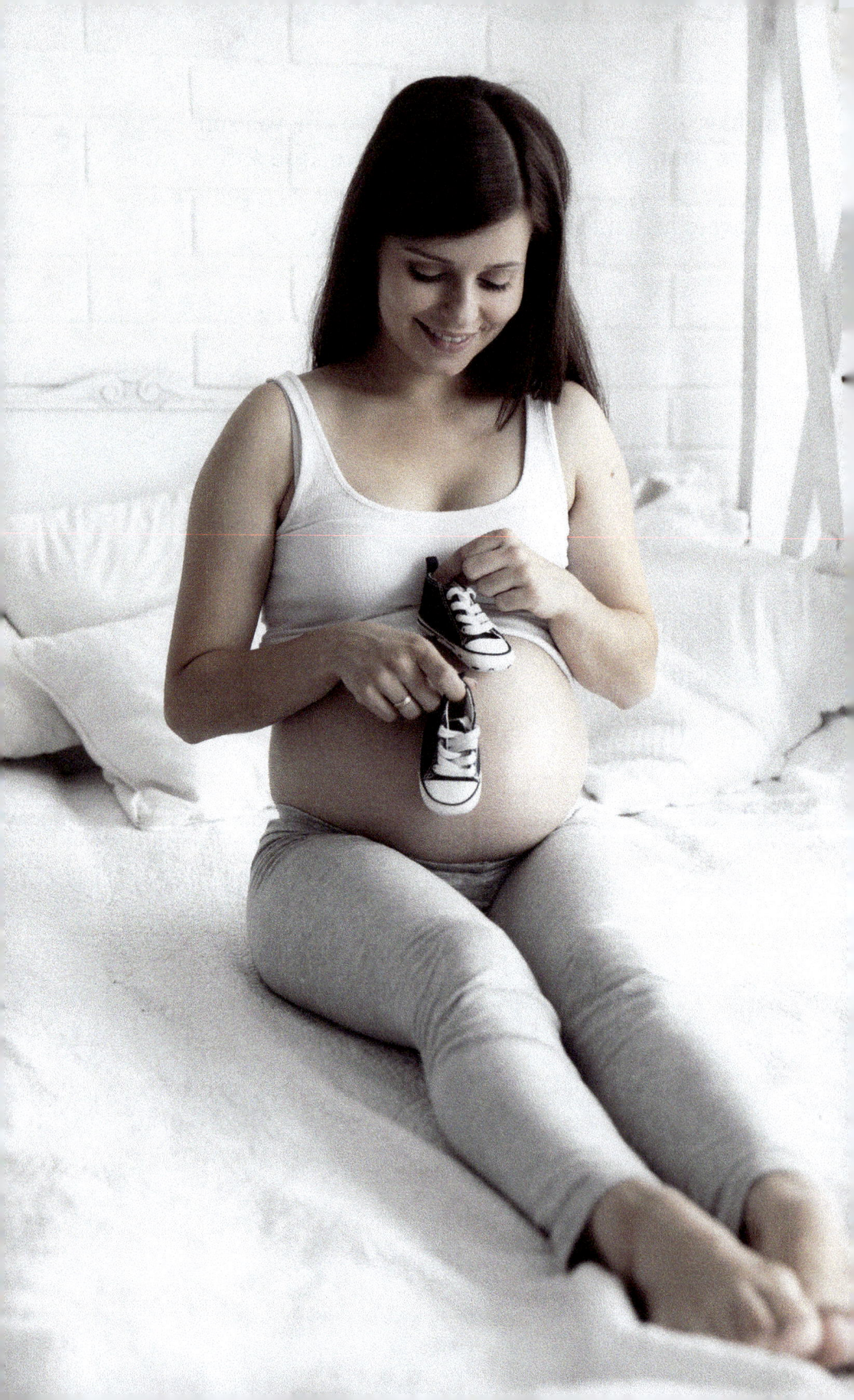

# Chapter 26: How Do I Lose Weight After Giving Birth?

New mothers usually despair for their pre-pregnancy body. They feel ashamed of their weight gain. Post-pregnancy weight gain is exceptionally natural, and there is nothing to be ashamed of. Just keep a positive frame of mind. You have made a baby; you are very powerful. Any kind of weight loss requires a mindset and effort.

So, in the last part, I have already discussed a postpartum ayurvedic diet for a new mom that not only helps in rejuvenation, but also helps in weight loss. I followed that same diet plan and was back to my pre-pregnancy weight just after six months. Of course, I followed exercise, yoga and even meditation.

First, let's talk about the science of burning fat. Postpartum our body needs a good number of vitamins, minerals, antioxidants etc. to function. So, if we consume fewer calories, but the diet is nutrient deficient, than our bodies will not burn fat as energy because the body recognizes low nutrition as scarcity and will store fat instead of burning.

When we eat solid, nourishing, and wholesome food high in nutrition, the body assumes that it is safe, and it releases its fat stores to be used as energy. This information really helped me in understanding the whole weight loss process.

- So, the first thing that I did for weight loss was drinking a lot of boiled herb-infused water that I discussed earlier. Whenever I felt hungry, I would drink water first and then wait for some time. If I still feel hungry, I'll eat, but most of the time I feel full. So, it was just tiredness, not hunger. Because somewhere I had read, we generally confuse tiredness with hunger. Being a new mom, you will always feel tired because of the lack of sleep and proper rest, so if you feel hungry drink a big glass of water and eat some fruit. It works when you are trying to lose weight.

- Secondly, I used to breastfeed, so naturally, my abdomen was shrinking. But we must understand that we cannot give on nutrition. Besides breastfeeding makes your body burn calories, which helps you lose weight. Just be patient, you will be surprised at how much weight you lose naturally while breastfeeding.

**Tips:**

- Do not skip meals. With a new baby, several new moms ignore eating, but if you do not eat, you will have a lesser amount of energy, and it will not assist you to lose weight. Eat 5 to 6 meals a day, with healthy snacks in between rather than three larger meals.

- Always eat a high fiber nutritious diet—snack on healthy fruits, vegetables, and nuts. Keep yourself away from any refined sugary stuff because you will end up feeling tired very quickly and you will also lose on your weight loss goal. I ate a very light but very nutritious diet, which made me heal promptly and even helped me in losing weight.

- Do not go on a crash diet or fad diet that limits a certain type of food and nutrients. They will probably make you drop some weight at first but will come back with a bang. It is never sustainable also.

- Drink plenty of herb-infused, boiled water.

- Take rest properly and try to get sleep, as much as possible, because it helps in losing weight.

- Join a post-pregnancy weight loss support group.

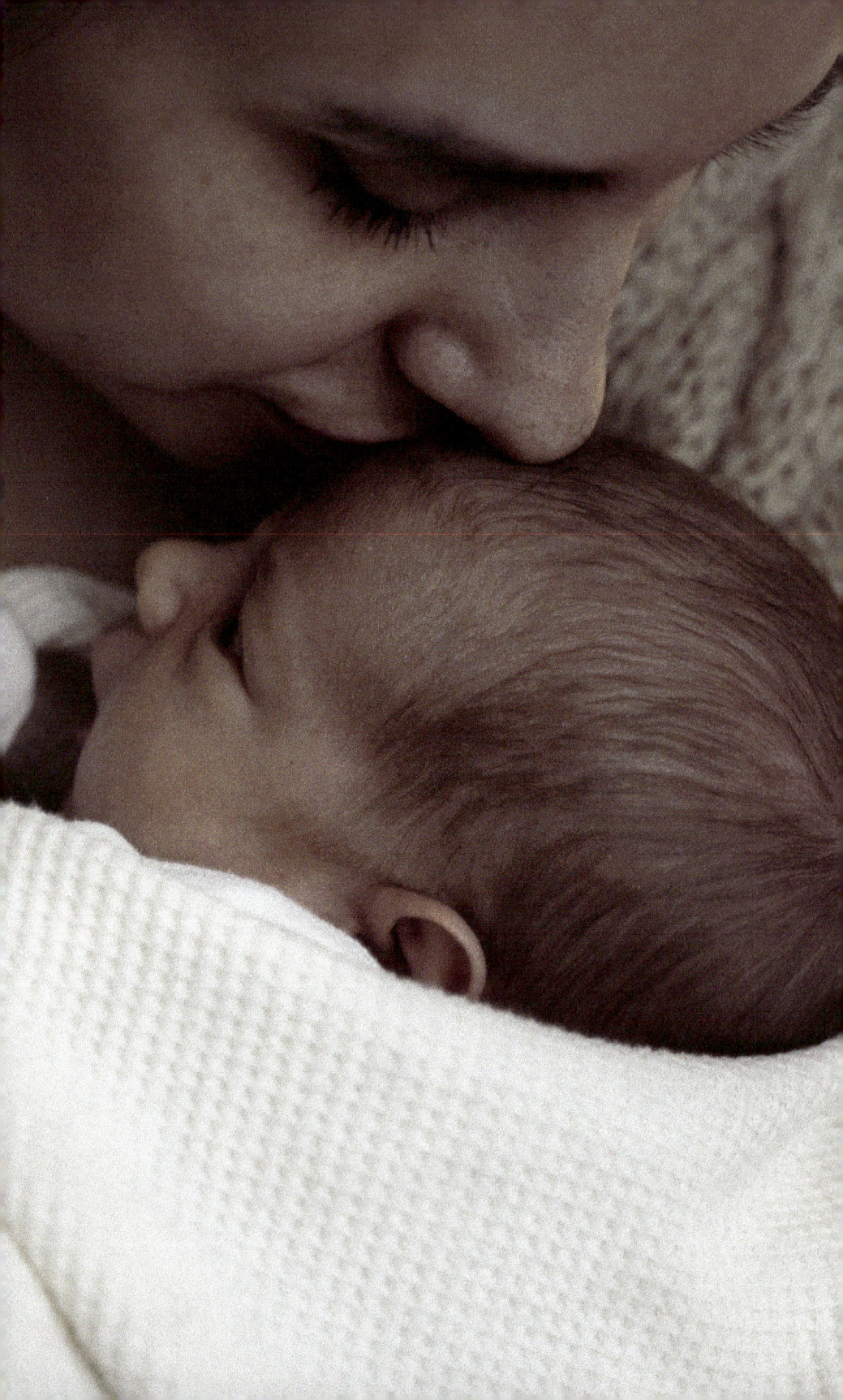

# Chapter 27: Extra Care for a Cesarean Recovery

Even if you had a normal, uneventful pregnancy, your chance of having a cesarean is nearly one in four. Since 25 percent of women will have a cesarean in the United States, you need to be aware of your risks.

The exercises for a vaginal birth are also applicable to cesarean recovery. The focus on your breathing will be stressed, because after surgery there are some complications that you are more likely to experience, like blood clots and breathing difficulties. Breathing deeply can help prevent these.

It is also imperative that you begin walking as soon as you can. Your intestines will be sluggish after surgery, and walking will help increase the movement of your intestines, peristalsis, as well as decrease the time of your recovery. It also helps avoid some complications of postpartum.

Getting up for the first time after a cesarean surgery is not fun. Find a pillow or other soft object to clutch to your abdomen. You might feel in the same way as you are going to spurt or that your organs will drop out. This is standard and will pass rapidly, predominantly the further you get up and get moving.

After a cesarean, you will also want to limit how much weight you lift or carry. A good rule is to carry nothing heavier than your baby for a few weeks. You will also want to minimize the amount of stair climbing you do. Set up a makeshift nursery downstairs. This prevents you from being isolated in your room and yet also keeps you from taking forty treks upstairs for diapers.

### *The First Few Days After Surgery*

Having a surgical birth can leave you physically exhausted and in pain. Keep in mind that you are not only experiencing the normal postpartum occurrences, such as changes in hormones and bleeding, but you are also recovering from major abdominal surgery.

The exercises for the first few days after surgery really focus on the prevention of complications. Learning to breathe after an abdominal incision is not as easy as it sounds. However, the more deep breathing you do, the less likely you are to have complications. As you hold your incision with your hands or brace it with a pillow, inhale. Put enough pressure or support on your abdomen so that you don't feel your incision will open. Do this frequently in the first few days to help prevent problems with your recovery.

In addition, try these exercises:

### Walk

The first few times you get up to walk after surgery are likely to be slow and painful. Use a pillow or your hands to brace your incision. While it may feel like your organs are going to fall out, you have many layers of stitches inside your body, as well as external stitches or staples. It doesn't sound like a lot of fun but getting up and walking will speed your recovery. On the first day or two, you will need someone to help you. By the second postpartum day, you will probably be asked to walk around the postpartum floor or nurses' station several times a day.

### Abdominal Tightening

As you lie in bed, or on the floor, have your knees bent and your feet flat on the floor. Tighten your buttocks and press your lower back into the bed or floor. As you inhale, imagine pulling your stomach down through your back to the floor or bed. Hold for up to five seconds. You can repeat this up to ten times.

### Leg Slides

Lie down on your back, and bend your right leg up, leaving your left leg flat on the bed, toes up. Slide your right leg down to rest next to your left leg. Slide it back up to the bent position again. Repeat this exercise five to ten times. Then repeat it with your left leg. If you're more comfortable, try holding a pillow over your incision while you do this exercise.

### The Second Week After Surgery

As your recovery progresses you will be able to do more and more. Do keep in mind that you have had major abdominal surgery, in addition to the joys of postpartum and new motherhood. Be sure to ask for help around the house and remember to allow others to do what they can. The less you do now, the faster you will heal completely.

These more advanced exercises can be tried in the second week postpartum:

### Pelvic Roll

Lie on your back with your feet together. Your knees should be bent. As you hold your knees together, bring them up toward your chest. Roll them to your right side. Slowly roll them to your left side. This is a gentle rocking motion. You should avoid any jerking or bouncing while doing this. If this exercise pulls on your incision, stop doing it immediately. Repeat this up to ten times on each side.

### Abdominal Strengthening

Lie down on your back with your feet together and knees slightly bent. Crisscross your arms over your abdomen, grabbing your waist on the opposite side.

As you lift your head, pull your arms together, thus pulling your stomach muscles toward each other. Try to imagine that you have an apple under your chin to ensure proper head alignment during this exercise. Don't go too far up; your shoulders should barely leave the ground when doing this. Hold the pose for three to five seconds and then relax your head and arms to the original starting position. Repeat this exercise up to five times.

During the first two weeks' postpartum from a cesarean delivery, you should refrain from walking the stairs more than about once a day. You should not drive your car, and keep in mind that you should not attempt to lift anything heavier than your baby.

### The Third Week After Surgery

By now you probably feel much better, though you still have some lingering pain and tension. Be sure to listen to your body and watch your incision. Add exercises slowly to the last week's exercises as you build your body back up:

### Pelvic Tilt

After about two weeks, you can begin to do your pelvic tilts. Assume an all-fours position, on your hands and knees. Think of holding your back in its natural alignment. Then tuck only your pelvis in, bringing your pubic bone toward your neck. Be sure to move only your pelvis. If it helps, have someone hold your pelvis so that you can learn to isolate this area. Later this exercise can be done in different positions. You need to do two sets of up to ten repetitions of the pelvic tilts. Later, you can add more to each set of repetitions.

The area of your incision may feel numb. Some women report that this numbness lasts for years, if not permanently. You might also feel like there is itching below the skin. This is also normal. The surgery requires that muscles and therefore nerves be cut, thus causing this damage. Always tell your doctor or midwife if your incision is bothering you.

After the beginning exercises of breathing and abdominal tightening of the first few days, you will slowly begin to feel better. Your recovery will usually not be as fast as that of your vaginal-birth counterparts, but you can affect the length of time you take to recover by not doing too much.

Once you've been given the go-ahead for exercising, you will want to pay particular attention to your abdominal muscles. If you had a low transverse or bikini incision, you would not have as severe of an abdominal problem than if you required a classical or vertical incision.

## Goal Setting: Now and Then

It is important to establish both short-term and long-term goals as part of your weight-loss plan. Short-term goals help you reach long-term goals by acting as small steps and keeping you motivated throughout the process. Short-term goals can help change behaviors and keep you motivated. Your goals should deal with specific problems, such as the need to eat more vegetables, and should be specific about what, where, when, and how of your planned changes. In other words, get yourself an action plan.

Short-term goals, such as drinking 64 ounces of water each day, can help change behaviors. Be specific about how you will reach your goal. It is too vague to simply say, "I will drink more water." This does not give you any specific action to work on. On the other hand, the statement, "I will buy a 32-ounce water bottle and fill it up and drink it twice a day" is specific enough that you can measure each day whether you have achieved your goal.

Short-term goals, such as a class reunion, can also help motivate you through your weight-loss process, but make sure you line up another goal as soon as that event is over to keep you going. A specific event should not be your final or long-term goal. Make your long-term goals more than just weight loss. Make them goals that will emerge from the weight loss, such as getting healthy, defining a positive self-image, taking better care of your children, having more energy, improving the quality of your life, eating better, and enjoying physical activity.

## One Step at a Time

Work on a few behaviors at a time, and once you have accomplished those, move on to a few more. Trying to bite off more than you can chew can be overwhelming as well as discouraging. Once you accomplish a short-term goal, move on to the next. A feeling of accomplishment can be a great motivational tool.

Here's an example:

Long-Term Goal: Improve my health risk factors.

Short-Term Goal: Eat breakfast every day.

Action Plan: Buy healthy breakfast foods to have on hand and get up fifteen minutes early to make time for breakfast.

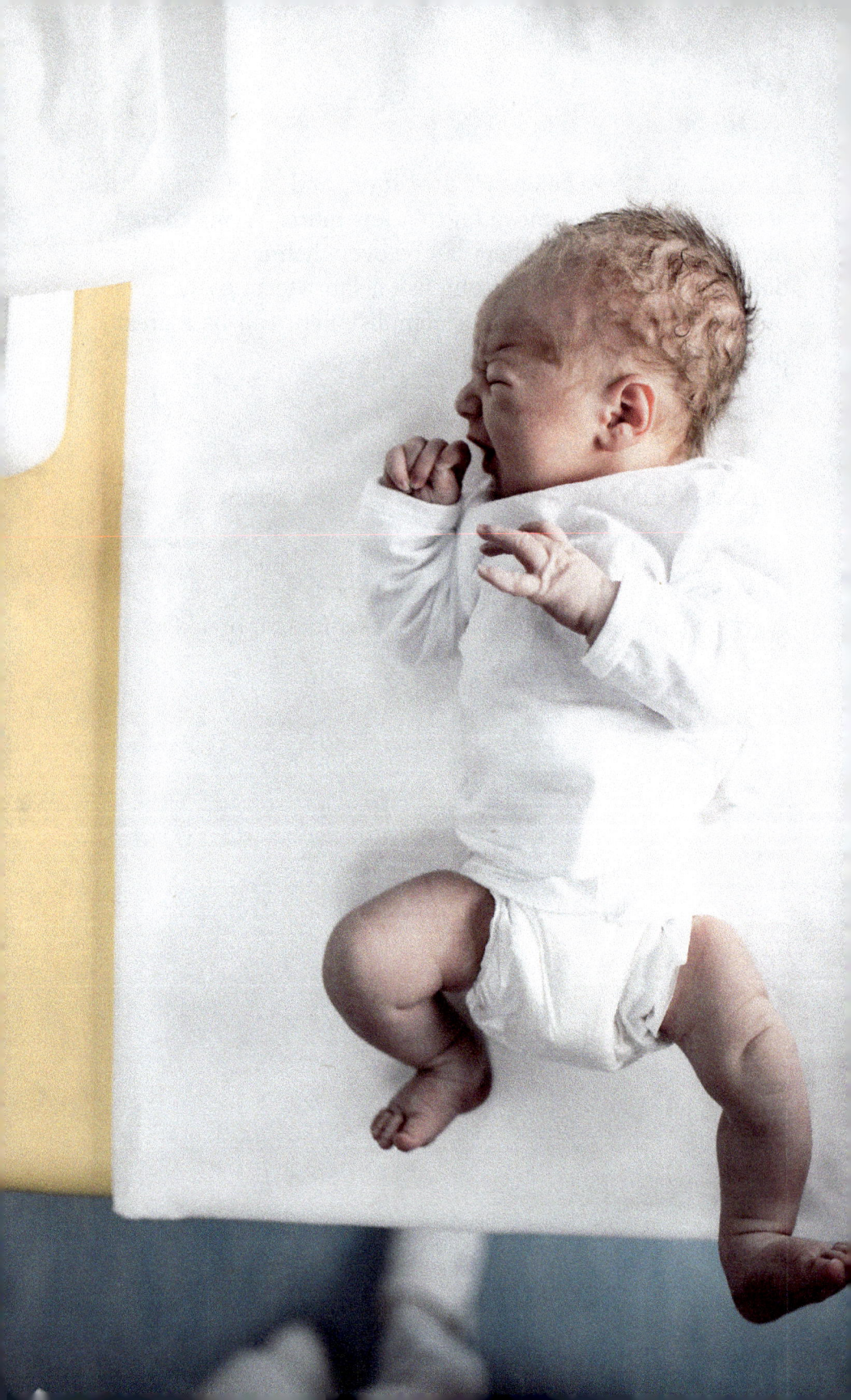

# Chapter 28: Growth and Development of the Baby

O nce your baby is here, you may start to wonder what is normal in terms of his or her growth and development. Know that every baby is different and your baby being a little bit behind of the average is not something to cause alarm, but let's take a look at what you most likely can expect in your baby's first year of life.

In those first couple of weeks of life you will probably notice some fluctuation in your baby's weight. Do not panic; this is perfectly normal. When your baby is first weighed in after birth you will likely be surprised as to how big your little baby is. This initial weigh in is known as the birth weight. Most of the time, your baby will lose a considerable amount of that birth weight within the first few days of life. Continue weekly pediatrician visits or check ins until your baby works back up to that initial birth weight to be sure that he or she is eating sufficiently and has not gotten sick.

As early as three weeks old your baby may start experiencing growth spurts. A lot of parents find that they are throwing out a considerable amount of newborn clothes with your baby outgrowing clothes before he or she even gets a chance to wear them! You will know that your baby is going through a growth spurt if he or she suddenly is wanting food more often and in greater quantity. For breastfeeding moms, you probably have just now gotten to the point where your baby is not demanding food every hour or two, but suddenly he or she is back to suckling hourly. Do not worry- this demanding feeding schedule will only last a couple of days- until your baby's next growth spurt that is!

By six weeks old you may start noticing that your baby is finally getting on some sort of schedule. It's okay if he or she is still a little inconsistent, but at this point you may want to start looking for advice from your doctor (or possibly family members) about how to get your baby on a more normal sleeping schedule. Do not worry if it takes a little longer for your baby though because every child is different.

By two months old your baby will likely be getting ready to start rolling over, reaching for toys, and maybe even sitting. By three months your baby will most definitely be on a more regular feeding and sleeping schedule. Most babies start teething around four months, but some will begin as early as three and others as late as twelve.

At six months your baby will start mastering what is known as the pincer grasp: grabbing small objects with the thumb and forefinger. Around seven months your baby will likely be clapping, pointing, and waving. A true personality is developing in your baby now. Most babies begin crawling around eight months, so if you have not already baby proofed your house now would be the time. By nine months your little crawler will become a climber! Be sure to keep a careful watch on your baby around stairs because he or she is going to want to climb them. Most babies will start walking anywhere between nine and eighteen months, so you may want to start shoe shopping fairly soon.

Again, keep in mind that every child is unique in terms of developmental milestones. If you are concerned whether or not your baby is behind, consult your doctor before you start to worry.

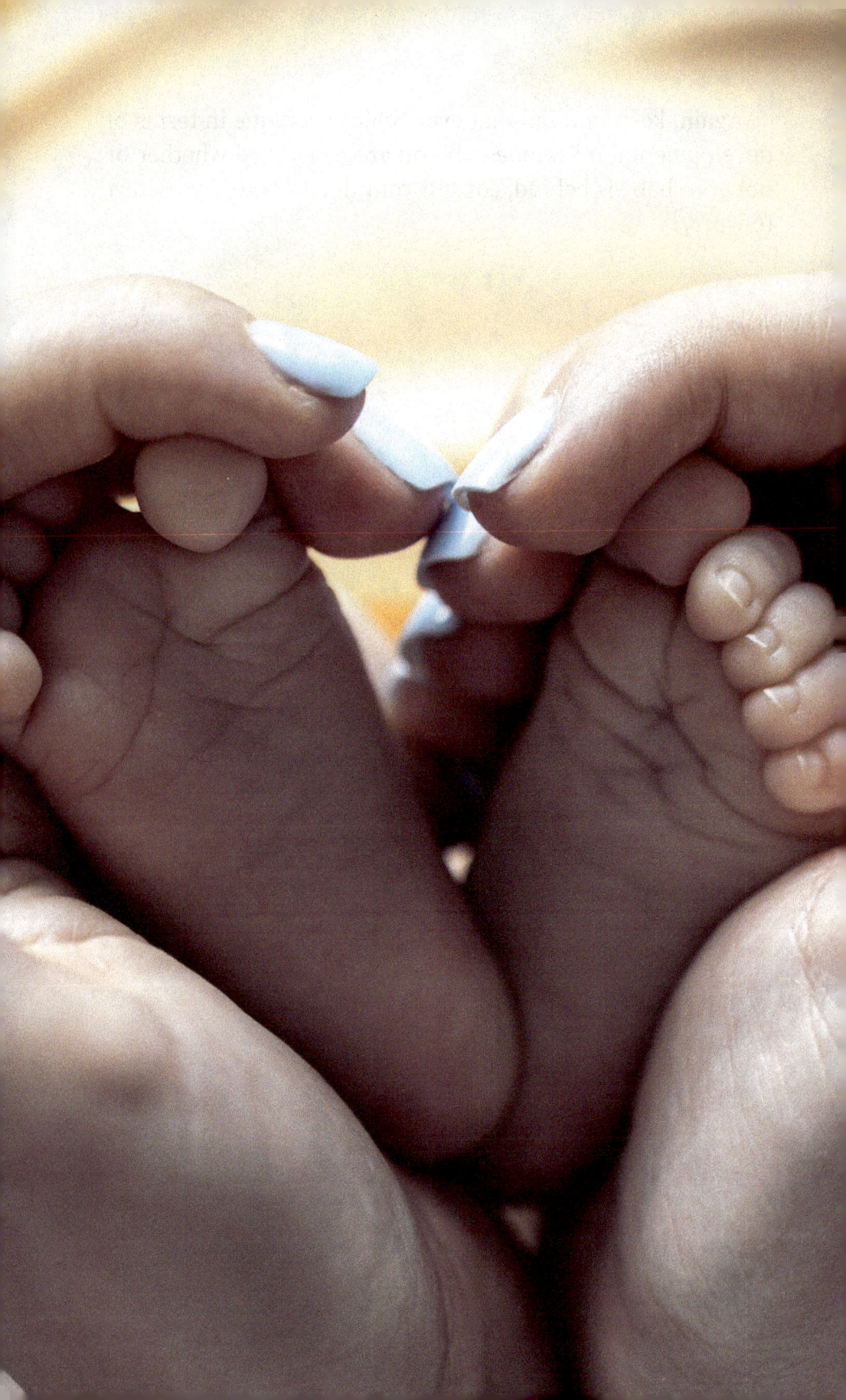

# Chapter 29: Common Question on Feeding and Caring of Your Newborn

**Q. How do I care for my baby's umbilical cord stump, and when will it fall off?**

Each care practitioner might tell you different things, but the general rule of thumb with umbilical cord care is to keep it dry. As gross as it sounds, this is a piece of flesh that is dying and will eventually fall off. If the cord gets goopy or smelly, you can take a cotton swab and clean the base with rubbing alcohol or hydrogen peroxide. The process of it falling off can take anywhere from two days to two weeks. If the skin becomes inflamed and red around the base of the cord, let your care provider know.

**Q. Is this normal? What is going on with my baby's poop?**

Immediately following the birth of your baby, you can expect to see a black, tarry poop called meconium. Your baby is born with this poop already in their intestinal tract and passes this at birth or soon after. There should be at least one meconium poop in the first 24-hour period. As this poop transitions from the black tarry substance, you will see it range from brown to green to yellow. If you're breastfeeding, once your milk is fully in, you will start to notice this poop turn into a mustard yellow with some seed-like specks in it. The poop should remain that color until solid foods or formula is introduced.

If you see green poop consistently, it could be an imbalance of your hindmilk and foremilk. You can seek lactation help on how to remedy this with ease. If you are formula feeding, your baby's poop will be more of a pasty consistency that is brown—and it can change from a more yellow-based brown to a more green-based brown.

### Q. How often should my baby pee and poop?

For the first few days, the general rule of thumb is that baby should produce the same number of wet and poopy diapers as the days since birth, so one wet and one poopy diaper in the first 24 hours, two wet and two poopy diapers in the second 24 hours, and so on. Typically, by day four, your milk has fully transitioned from colostrum and the size of the baby's stomach has grown, and from here on out, it's normal to see five to six wet diapers per day and three to four poopy diapers per day (and sometimes many more). Some babies also poop less, and that is still within normal limits. If you have any concerns, contact your pediatrician or a lactation specialist if you are breastfeeding. Formula-fed babies tend to poop less frequently than breast milk–fed babies because it is a heavier protein and moves through the intestines more slowly. In the beginning, they poop up to three to four times daily, but it isn't uncommon after the first few weeks to have them go longer between poops, sometimes up to seven days. As long as your baby's poop isn't formed like hard little pellets, you likely don't have to worry about constipation—but contact your care provider if you are concerned or if your baby seems uncomfortable.

## Q. What do I need to know about caring for and cleaning my baby's penis?

This will differ depending on whether your baby is circumcised or intact.

### Circumcision Care

Typically, the head (glans) of the circumcised penis is covered with gauze and petroleum jelly until the incision has healed to protect it from exposure to feces. Be sure to ask the care provider who performed the circumcision their recommendations on the proper care and cleaning for your child's circumcised penis.

### Intact Foreskin Care

For the care of an intact penis, there isn't much to do. The head of the penis (glans) is meant to be an internal organ, and the foreskin protects it. At this stage of development, there is a membrane between the foreskin and the glans that keeps the foreskin from retracting; this is normal. DO NOT retract the foreskin or let any care provider do so; the foreskin will naturally start to retract on its own between the ages of three and six years. Simply wipe away any debris that might be on the penis.

## Q. What do I need to know about caring for my baby's vulva and vagina?

One of the most shocking things to parents is that it is normal for a newborn's vulva to produce a white, thick discharge and even small blood-tinged discharge in the first few days. The baby received a hormonal boost at the end of the pregnancy, and these hormones can produce what is colloquially known as "first menstruation." Rest assured—this is totally normal and usually goes away in about a day or two. As for cleaning, there is no need to enter the vagina. Just take a wet cloth or wipe and gently remove any debris on the vulva. It's also a good idea to begin the practice of wiping from front to back, which you'll want to eventually teach your child to do during potty training, too.

### Q. What are some quick tips for newborn hygiene that I need to know?

Newborn Baths

Giving newborns baths is a little like bathing a wiggling, wet fish—it's hard! Be sure to take your time, have everything you need right next to you, and be prepared for possible tears, maybe from both of you. Laying a towel down in the tub or sink is also helpful in minimizing slipperiness. My (Lindsey's) favorite time with my own new babies was taking baths together. You can even add herbs to the bath—which could help with your healing, if you had a vaginal birth, and baby's umbilical cord healing as well.

Trimming Baby's Nails

Again, this is not an easy task. With newborns the easiest way to trim their nails is to file them down. Their nails are so thin that sometimes even tearing them to the side or biting them off is easier than trying to cut them. A good time to try this is while they are eating or sleeping.

Clearing The Nasal Passages

Newborns typically keep their nasal passages clear on their own, but if you're noticing extra snot, the best product on the market to keep them clear is the Nose Frida. (Don't let the description gross you out!) If your baby has boogers, you won't be the first parent to pick your baby's nose. Another good option is to use a cool-mist humidifier in the room where the baby sleeps.

## Q. What are the symptoms of and treatment for newborn jaundice?

The main signs and symptoms of newborn jaundice are yellowing of the eyes and skin. Jaundice typically is first visible in the whites of the eyes and then moves to the face, into the trunk of the body, and next into the extremities. Your pediatrician or your care provider will assess your newborn, and if the jaundice is severe enough, your baby might be hospitalized under UV lights for treatment. Frequent nursing and indirect sunlight for 15-minute increments, three times a day, can also help move the bilirubin out of your baby's system, lessening the need for medical treatment.

## Q. What do I need to know about newborn thrush?

Receiving IV antibiotics in labor can greatly increase the chances of newborn thrush. Thrush is basically a yeast infection of the mouth, nipples, and sometimes diaper area. If you have thrush, you will usually experience burning, red nipples that stay this way between feeds. You might also notice a white, milky substance that coats the baby's mouth but doesn't wipe away. Thrush is not fun to have and can be tricky to treat. Since yeast thrives off sugar, first things first are cutting sugar from your diet. There are prescription and over-the-counter anti-fungal medications that can be used to treat thrush. If you think either you or your baby is experiencing thrush, seek assistance from a lactation specialist.

## Q. Do newborns have a typical schedule I should follow?

Not really. A better word than the schedule is rhythm. You will learn your baby's rhythm, and it will ebb and flow as the days change. Typically, you will be nursing everyone to three hours over a 24-hour period. You're teaching each other, so set your expectations low and give yourself a lot of grace. We recommend the Taking Cara Babies newborn class (TakingCaraBabies.com) if you are someone who wants some semblance of a schedule.

## Q. How many hours of sleep should my baby get?

Babies sleep a lot in the newborn phase, but every baby is different, so don't set a certain expectation. The average newborn sleeps eight to nine hours a day and eight hours at night, which leaves just a few awake hours to feed, poop, and maybe eye gaze and coo with parents. Take advantage of naps, even though it sounds like a lot; if you aren't sleeping while they are, the broken sleep at night might catch up with you.

**Q. My baby hiccups a lot. Do I need to treat their hiccups?**

Hiccups are normal. Chances are if your baby hiccupped a lot in utero, they would hiccup a lot on the outside, too. There is no need to treat the hiccups, but if your baby is fussy and you're breastfeeding, you might consider eliminating top allergens (dairy, gluten, eggs) from your diet to see if what you're passing through your milk might be upsetting their tummy.

**Q. My baby's skin is breaking out. What should I do?**

Nothing. Baby acne is very common in the first two to four weeks of life, although some babies can get it later than four weeks. There's no firm understanding of what causes baby acne, though some believe it to be a result of your hormones from pregnancy. It will go away on its own without any treatment.

**Q. What is cradle cap, and how do I treat it?**

Cradle cap is a dandruff-like, crusty scale that sometimes happens on the top of your baby's head. It is usually caused by an overactive oil-producing gland. It is reported that up to 70 percent of newborns have experienced this by the age of three months. While you don't have to do anything to treat cradle cap, you can mix a carrier oil with a gentle anti-fungal essential oil like lavender or geranium and softly massage it into your baby's scalp.

### Q. How can I tell if my newborn is hungry?

If you watch your newborn, you will learn their hunger cues. Crying is the last sign of hunger, so look for signs of your baby starting to root (make sucking motions when their lips or cheeks are touched). They will bring their hands to their mouth, bob their head up and down, and step their feet. If you respond when you start noticing these signs, you will likely avoid latching or trying to bottle feed a frantic baby, which makes it so much easier.

# Chapter 30: Baby's Transition to Earth Side

The mother's experience of birth is well documented and observed. The newborn's experience is barely mentioned except for a few specific studies on cord blood transfer and maybe some books on natural birth rituals (such as lotus birthing). But newborns have an experience as well. It would be absurd to say they don't, as they are clearly people with consciousness whose environment drastically changes. In classical philosophy it has long been noted that children's experiences shape them in disposition and mental state – even those experiences they were seemingly too young to remember. But the body remembers. They may not have the mental processing ability to verbalize what happened, but it can still affect them. Some forms of hypnotherapy and even regular therapy occasionally make a tie back to the birth experience. So, what does the newborn experience? In a natural birth, the baby releases hormones that signal they are ready to come out. These hormones start contractions and a host of other processes to ready baby and mother for birth.

Baby starts feeling strong cushy pulses around them – similar to when you squeeze a water balloon. You can't hurt something that is inside because of the water cushion, but you can squeeze the balloon pretty strongly and effectively. They start to rotate and get pushed along from a soft, cushy pod headfirst into a hard, boney tunnel that squeezes their head and face as they keep getting pushed. They slowly slip, twist, and inch along the tight tunnel until they come out into a chilly, bright, dry, noisy environment where for the first time ever they feel stronger sensations on their skin than just amniotic fluid. Gone is the steady echoing heartbeat, the transference of air and food, the easy elimination. The baby will now hear the sounds of the world much more clearly and loudly, transition to breathing air, feel hunger for the first time, feel cold, and feel touch. All the senses will be used in an entirely different way for the first time in their lives. Regulating environment and even emotions are all their own now. No more shared hormones or feelings. From a different perspective that may be easier to envision, imagine you are floating in a closed relaxation pod. The door is closed, you feel weightless, you recently ate a wonderful meal and do not need the bathroom, soothing music is on, the light is very dim, and the atmosphere is pleasant. Then there is a lot of jerking around, maybe new noises, your water may be drained, you may be pulled, the pod door thrown open. There is cheering, yelling, bright lights, and you are deftly, roughly handled and placed far from the pod, perhaps you even feel sharp pain for the first time in your life, have your vision blurred. You are in shock and disoriented, you go with the flow of what is happening to you and wait for a break to settle. You may not ever again feel any of the sensations you had in the pod. You may not receive comfort or acknowledgement to what happened. You may not be comforted in any way. A baby can have a wide range of experiences. Imagine yourself in the pod. How would you like to emerge? Be kind to your baby. You may not be able to regulate every single aspect of their emergence. You may not even be able to regulate any of it. But you can be thereafter.

What happens after? In a normal, undisturbed birth, the mother and baby have a slight pause right after the baby comes out. This is the "birth pause." It is when the mother and baby stop to take a moment and process what happened. They may not even look at each other yet. It is a peaceful moment of processing. Then, the mother lifts her baby up onto her chest and watches as the baby does the breast crawl. If it is chilly, they both may be covered by a light blanket. The baby knows his mother's smell and is drawn to the nipple, which darkens toward the end of pregnancy specifically for this purpose – to be visible to the baby. Colostrum comes only in droplets at a time at first and milk doesn't normally come until day three or so, but baby is on the breast to signal that they are here, on the outside. There are receptor glands on the mother's nipples that receive information from the baby's saliva and the milk adjusts to the order the baby placed. Nipple stimulation as well as the baby's motion on the mother's abdomen of crawling up to the breast both help contract the uterus and expel the placenta. Once the baby is on the mom – either rooting, smelling, latched on, or sleeping – the "golden hour" begins. This is the hour immediately post-birth when both mother and baby process what just happened, when they connect and discover each other's presence on the exterior. Mothers are drawn strongly to the smell of their newborns – especially their heads.

The smell of baby starts up a cascade of oxytocin and bonding hormones. Oxytocin is a natural hormone that serves many purposes: it expels the placenta, contracts the uterus, creates feelings of calm, and helps with relaxing so milk comes in faster. The baby, skin to skin with the mother, is back to hearing the familiar heartbeat, being surrounded by familiar smells, hearing the voice they are used to, and a touch that they connect with.

Many studies have proven the strong mother/baby bond that exists. A mother's presence even in the same room can lower the baby's stress hormones and regulate their sleep. The closer they are together the higher the benefits. A mother's breasts can change the temperature up or down up to two degrees to regulate the baby's body temperature, breathing, heartbeat, hormones, pain levels, and even digestion with close contact. This is all essential information because normal newborn procedures are usually done in this time. Then the wiped, clothed, pricked, and otherwise handled baby is handed back to the mother (or placed in a nursery for contact with the mom at some later time).

Unless there is a life or death emergency, everything for both the mom and her baby can be done with the duo held together, undisturbed. There is also no need for any procedure to be done at this time since it can be just as well done at a later time. When choosing your provider and location, keep in mind how you want this experience to be for your baby, as procedures and protocols can vary significantly based on those choices. Also, educate yourself on the risks, benefits, and alternatives to all procedures.

In keeping with the gentle newborn experience, what do you truly need to welcome a baby into the world? A mother and a warm blanket, perhaps some diapers. The first three months of a newborn's life are called the "fourth trimester." This is when the baby fully finishes transitioning from womb to life earth side. During this time, the baby's needs are still roughly the same as in the womb – warmth, gentle motion, closeness to their mother, breastmilk, and elimination on demand.

# Chapter 31: Hypnobirthing for Mom and Baby

### *Hypnobirthing for a Healthier Mother and Baby*

Medicine has enabled humanity to achieve and maintain optimum health. Unfortunately, the introduction of new drugs is showing its consequences even in a healthy body. Drug-assisted delivery is questioned because of the use of narcotics. Nowadays the use of hypnotic childbirths for a healthy baby is not popular for mums.

Once ether was found women gave birth to the natural way. Although its advances culminated in anesthesia, some people often opted to give birth to the natural process. It became widespread during the 1960s and 1970s. Now the process of giving birth is resurfacing as a safer way.

Medical interventions were shown to have unwanted effects on mother and baby. Drugs used during treatment have side effects that present a threat to both mother and child. The analgesic and anesthesia used could worsen the baby's delivery.

Drugs such as Demerol and Stanol trigger mother and child to suffer from respiratory depression. Nubian sedates the kid when it is born and causes low scores of APGAR.

Epidurals may be able to delay distribution. That can proceed to a more complicated medical procedure. A cesarean section is an expensive, large abdominal procedure. It weakens the mother's uterine defenses, which may crack during her successive pregnancies. It can also lead in vacuum extraction or distribution of forceps. Extraction of the vacuum will trigger hemorrhage that is fatal for the infant. A medical tool will be used during forceps childbirth to remove the infant from the birth canal. Forceps will leave marks on your baby's head that he / she must hold until he / she is adult.

A hypnotic method was created to help the mother get a painless and comfortable delivery in reaction to the increasing rate of natural childbirth. It is one of the strategies used to manage pain during a natural childbirth.

To some, it's unlikely to have a painless treatment without drugs. How will hypnosis help during these painful contractions? Medicated aided delivery was the standard method of giving birth.

We have been taught in our society to look upon childbirth as a very painful process. We see this on TV and in movies. We are learning it from family and friends personal accounts. When we grow up, we perceive childbirth to be traumatic, which is one of the reasons why it is. childbirth hypnosis is not like what you see on tv or in film. Mothers are not likely to go through a state of trance. This is not going to help the kid get out. If the mind of the mother wanders or looks into space who will drive the baby out?

There were a lot of misunderstandings about hypnosis. More often than not, manipulating another human is synonymous with some magic trick. Television shows have shown us it's used to humiliate someone else. Anyone can get hypnotized, too. Contrary to popular belief it is actually easier to hypnotize strong minded people.

The hypnotherapist's not going to control the moms. They act only as a reference while distributing. The mother will be the only one able to enter a hypnotic trance. Even, she can go in and out as she wants.

Hypnosis is about keeping the mind calm and primed. The subconscious may be conditioned to adjust how we feel pain and interpret it. This may raise the pain threshold, in effect. Without any drugs, you can alleviate the discomfort. You will train the mind to experience pain as nothing but distress, through effective self-hypnosis.

There are workshops offered to educate the mother about Hypnobirthing. There are also instructional audio CD's online. These courses, however, will have no impact if the mother has made up her mind that it won't work. Hypnosis is about allowing use of the subconscious inside. As long as the mom is open to new ideas, she can have a positive mind with an effective self-hypnosis.

Hypnotic childbirths can be used for a healthy baby and mother. It will encourage the mother to have a calm, awake and alert birthing experience. Without the influence of drugs, the baby will come out robust. When home, the mother will heal quicker and easier to care for her infant. It's all in the attitude occasionally.

What you should learn about Childbirth Pain management in childbirth is natural, stable, and successful— and finishes with birth happiness. While labor pain management plays less of a role in the happiness of a mother with childbirth compared to the quality of the partnership with her job help and her ability to take part in decision making, it is an important topic.

Pain in childbirth is an almost common experience for women in childbearing. Nevertheless, birthing mothers view something distinctly. Nonetheless, most women require some kind of pain relief during childbirth. Techniques range from medications to natural methods, so attention should be provided well in advance of the various options open to you.

Non-pharmacological labor pain relief approaches are becoming more popular as moms, as well as pregnant women and nurses, become more conscious of the effectiveness of such strategies. Changing positions and breathing, warm water pools, yoga, and acupressure, alongside relaxing and Hypnobirthing, are gaining more interest in treating labor pain.

A longitudinal 2005 survey by Childbirth Connection found that 69 percent of birth mothers used at least one non-pharmacological tool to relieve pain and improve relaxation during their pregnancy. The calming exercises and adjustments of posture and behavior were most commonly employed, accompanied by stimulation, imagination, or hypnosis. Use hands-on methods such as acupuncture and labour acupressure, as many as one in five birthing mothers did. The vast majority of 91 per cent of mothers considered these two hands-on approaches to be very effective.

The effectiveness of these forms of pain relief is focused on the simplicity and ease of using them with no unique and costly equipment anywhere. This is in comparison to the extremely satisfactory level of job pain relief.

Strategies for relieving labor pain that are less widely employed include birthing balls, birth tub or shower, and aromatherapy. Only mothers who use these forms of pain relief usually view them as effective. Sadly, the need for special equipment or room restricts their use.

Labour is an exciting event that involves a lot of new sensations, particularly when you have your first infant. Those emotions are part of giving your baby life. No one needs to suffer during childbirth though. You are most likely to have a fulfilling birth experience by knowing what you can do, and how others can help you to avoid and alleviate labor pains.

### Hypno-Moms

The second boy is on his way. In reality, you're in your third trimester and have had vivid nightmares about the horrendous pain that heralded your firstborn's childbirth. You just wish there were some way to stop it. You might be able to trade in it for something less, yes, unpleasant. It is exactly this desire to avoid suffering that has prompted countless people to seek the hypnosis during childbirth.

Hypnosis has already been shown to function to relieve discomfort after injuries in fields such as dentistry and psychological counseling. It just makes sense that if this procedure can be used to reduce pain in one region it could do it for something as physically challenging as childbirth.

Childbirth hypnosis is typically a self-hypnosis and is the mother's conscious choice. No one else can bring you outside yourself under hypnosis at such a stressful time. Many mothers choose to have a hypnotherapist present to help achieve the self-hypnotic condition, but that hypnotherapist is merely a reference and cannot hypnotize the mother in fact.

The vast majority of the population can be hypnotized (about 90 percent), but the ability to truly believe in the efficacy in hypnosis of childbirth is essential to its effectiveness. Believe it or not, the greater your determination, the more stubborn you become, the harder it will be for you to reach the self-hypnotic condition in which you can experience a comfortable, pain-free childbirth.

Hypnosis in childbirth is a wonderful alternative to taking potentially harmful medications. This is also a reasonable option for women who have specific reactions to certain drugs. This ensures that your infant will not get these same medications.

In fact, there are many misconceptions and theories around hypnosis which just don't matter when coping with hypnosis in childbirth. Of starters, often people believe they can be persuaded to do things they wouldn't normally do or utter things they wouldn't normally say when they're hypnotized. This is simply not the case here, because an unknown person doesn't hypnotize you.

You practice self-hypnosis which is very similar to the way people calm down when they are extremely scared, frustrated, or distressed. You're not going to tell anyone any of your identities (or theirs you may be safeguarding). Suddenly, you are not going to have an impulse to "cluck" like a ham. You are always in full control of your body and emotions. At any moment you have the opportunity to get yourself out of the hypnotic state.

You're going to want to find a qualified hypnotherapist in your region to start helping you so you're happy on the day of childbirth. Most training sessions on childbirth hypnosis operate for about 6-7 hours and differ in size. There are also home-study courses available, so you don't need to try to find time to run once or twice a week to someone's school. Just use a reputable search engine and use phrases such as "hypnosis home study in childbirth" and you'll have a lot of options available.

The important point to remember is that if you choose to conceive using birth hypnosis, the delivery doesn't have to be traumatic or exhausting for you or your new baby. Many mothers who have used such methods of hypnosis rarely actually mention any discomfort at all. They've only got very happy, very vivid memories of this great day.

Your Mental Strength-Why is Your Flawless childbirth Visualized?

Visualization is a very powerful tool that can be used to build the ideal experience of childbirth. If you can't think about it - then how can you do it? You should take simple steps to help you achieve the precise birth you desire. Educate yourself first!

There's a lot to know about planning to bring a new life into this world-especially since this typical thing is mostly managed in our society by a highly medical community. The next move is to select the right careers. Only think of what you want for your birth! Spend some time determining what an optimal birth scenario would be for you and your relatives, and then choose a care provider that will help it.

Another stage sometimes ignored when planning for childbirth is the task of visualizing and getting the childbirth experience to fruition for yourself. Knew that many well-known athletes utilize imagination as part of their regular training programs to achieve the results they want? The brain knows nothing of the difference between a real and an imaginary one! Many Olympic athletes consider themselves to compete beautifully and win the gold medal. You can use the same methods that elite athletes use to get the outcome you want - a stunning, healthy birthing experience!

# Conclusion

Pregnancy is a time of excitement, anticipation, and preparation—it can also be a time of feeling uncomfortable and unsure of what comes next. If you can focus on the positive and at the very least know what to expect then you can make it through much easier. This is easier said than done sometimes but having a vision as you do know of what is common within the range of weeks can really help you to stay ahead of the game. The straightforward and honest approach is always much easier to allow you to move forward with a clear head.

Though you are going to likely feel some unpleasant symptoms this is all testament to the fact that baby is developing and growing properly. Try to remember that with each phase come some huge positives and some potential negatives. You may feel uncomfortable in the third trimester for example, but the baby will be here soon. You may struggle through the first trimester with exhaustion and even nausea, but for most that will be short lived. Everything that you feel is in the interest of this baby and making a smooth and happy environment for them.

The breakdown of these weeks is to show you not only what is going on with the baby, but also with you as the mother. You are more than just the vehicle for baby's development and so you must take good care of yourself as well. Try to get some rest whenever possible and really focus on what this is all about. This may be easier said than done but it can greatly help as you move forward in anticipation of baby's arrival.

Some phases may move very quickly, and some may seem to stand still in time, but they are all an important part of the process.

Know that you will get your body back, but it may take time. Once you get past the hump and you start to get some sleep again then you can start exercising when you feel up to it. You can also focus on proper diet and even getting some rest, which are all important to making yourself feel normal. Know that it will come in time and be patient. It took you nine months to put the weight on and so it won't come off overnight, so take your time and know that you will be back to your normal self in no time at all!

Your pregnancy will change and evolve with every week that you go through. You are going to feel wonderful things such as baby's kicks and that will overshadow the discomfort that you might feel in other areas. Try to remain calm and stay focused on what this is all about. Yes, your body is going to change a lot and it will get back to normal. In the meantime, though you get to experience something truly magical and that is the development of your new little bundle of joy. Pregnancy can be a miraculous time, so try to focus on all the wonderful positives and remember that any of the negatives will pass quickly and soon be a thing of the past before you even realize it.

www.ingramcontent.com/pod-product-compliance
Lightning Source LLC
Chambersburg PA
CBHW051719020426
42333CB00014B/1064